Ruth

DIET FOR LIFE

The New *Joyous* Way
to Permanent Slimness,
High Energy, Sexual Vigor,
Glowing Physical
and Mental Health
—and Added Youthful Years

Francine Prince

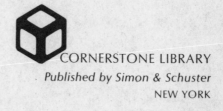

CORNERSTONE LIBRARY
Published by Simon & Schuster
NEW YORK

Copyright © 1981 by Francine Prince
All rights reserved
including the right of reproduction
in whole or in part in any form
Published by Cornerstone Library, Inc.
A Simon & Schuster Division of
Gulf & Western Corporation
Simon & Schuster Building
1230 Avenue of the Americas
New York, New York 10020

CORNERSTONE LIBRARY and colophon are
trademarks of Simon & Schuster, registered in
the U.S. Patent and Trademark Office.

Manufactured in the United States of America
10 9 8 7 6 5 4 3

Library of Congress Cataloging in Publication Data

Prince, Francine.
  Diet for life.

  Includes indexes.
  1. Diet. 2. Nutrition. 3. Reducing diets.
4. Low-fat diet. 5. Salt-free diet. I. Title.
RA784.P74   613.2   80–27837

ISBN 0–346–12496–4

To Norman Monath

For his foresight, his wisdom, and above all, for his warmth and kindness

Caution

This book is based on the experiences of myself and my husband, and on our studies of nutritional literature. It is not intended, nor should it be regarded, as medical advice. Before changing your diet, it would be prudent to first consult with your physician.

Contents

DIET
FOR LIFE

What the Diet for Life Can Do for You

It changed our lives. It could change yours.

It's a diet for the rest of your life, for the sake of your life.

It's a diet based on the joys of eating, of loving, of living.

The Saturday Evening Post called it:

A stunning breakthrough in diet cuisines. . . . Low-calorie, low-fat, low-saturated fat, low-cholesterol, no-sugar, no-salt, it's a gourmet cuisine for people of all ages.

Earl Ubell, health and science editor, CBS-TV News, added:

The food is excellent without grease or fat. And the salt-free bread beats most breads you can buy in a store. For my sweet tooth, the sherbet made with pineapple and egg white, no sugar added, outshines ice cream.

And Universal Press Syndicate concluded the Diet for Life:

. . . could add years to the average person's life. Mouthwatering!

The Diet for Life is a program for slimming down to your ideal weight—and doing it for the first two weeks without sacrificing a calorie.

It's a program for remaining at your ideal weight permanently—while expanding the joys of the table.

It's a program for staying healthy, and helping ward off nutrition-related diseases like heart attack, hypoglycemia, atherosclerosis, hypertension, and diabetes without recourse to drugs or disagreeable forms of therapy.

It's a program based on Dr. Norman Jolliffe's famous Prudent Diet, which, over many years of experiments, cut heart attack by an amazing 500 percent, and was effective against a long list of diseases.

It's a program based also on many of the sound nutritional guidelines approved by the American Medical Association, the American Heart Association, and the U.S. Departments of Agriculture and Health, Education, and Welfare.

In this book you'll learn everything you should know about nutrition, so you can make informed decisions about your most precious possession—your health.

Here is the practical, detailed information you've always wanted on salt and sugar, saturated and unsaturated fats, and cholesterol. Here are answers to your questions about yogurt, honey, fructose, bean sprouts, fiber, and health-food restaurants (you're in for some surprises).

Here is a complete rundown on the culinary and health-promoting uses of garlic and other herbs, and of spices. Here's a review of what vitamins and minerals can do for you mentally, as well as physically.

Here's an eating plan for staying at the peak of your energy all day long.

And because exercise is a vital element of the Diet for Life program, here's how the oldest, most natural, and the most joyous exercise in the world, walking, can tune up your body and heighten your spirits while helping to eliminate fatigue.

You'll find here a table of ideal weights, a list of the caloric and sodium content of healthful foods, a chart showing how your daily caloric requirement declines as you grow older, and a roster of low-sodium commercial foods that pass our taste test.

You'll find out how to calculate how many pounds of fat you'll lose each week on a reducing diet, and how many calories a day you need to keep your weight rock-steady on a maintenance diet.

You'll find health-conscious gourmet guides to the meat market, the fish market, the poultry market—and learn about the percentages of fats in the foods you buy there. You'll find data on the health values and the taste values of salad oils, and cooking fats and oils. You'll find out the truth about low-fat cheeses. You'll even find a surprising list of "high-cholesterol" foods you can live with—including shrimp.

You'll find out how other diets—including Tarnower's, Atkins', and Pritikin's—compare with the Diet for Life; and how the nutrient contents of each diet compare with the Federal Dietary Guidelines (the Diet for Life conforms most closely). You'll find out what's wrong with other diets nutritionally, and especially gastronomically.

There's no way you can stay on a reducing diet, then stick to a maintenance diet, unless the food is a constant source of delight. It *is* on the Diet for Life, and only on the Diet for Life. The proof came when my *The Dieter's Gourmet Cookbook: Delicious Low-Fat, Low-Cholesterol Cooking and Baking Recipes Using No Sugar or Salt!* broke sales records, and letters of praise flooded in from all over the nation.

"Your cookbook was a major discovery to me," one dieter wrote, "because we were so tired of eating tasteless food."

Another:

"I think you are a miracle. Your book is so unusual, so thorough, and so delightful that it is beyond my ability to do it justice. Now there is no reason for anyone to cook improperly. What a boon to mankind!"

And another:

"Congratulations for giving dieters who had to prepare uninteresting and almost unpalatable meals the chance to shine in the kitchen once more . . . and enjoy eating again. I am extolling this book to contacts from our family physician to our local health-food and specialty stores."

And a nurse wrote:

"Instead of flowers, I now give your book as a gift to heart patients."

Diet for Life is not a cookbook, although it does contain 115 *new* low-fat, low-cholesterol, no-sugar, no-salt cooking and baking recipes and variations, plus a chapter on how to convert your favorite recipes to Diet for Life-type recipes.

Diet for Life is not only for people on restricted diets. It's for all people who love life, and who want to get the most out of every minute through sparkling health of body and of mind.

Our diet not only restored my husband to peak vigor after a heart attack (the story is in Part 1), but also beautified our view of life. It slowed down our aging clock, and invigorated our sex life. It raised our capacities to work, to think, to succeed, to be happy—to live life to the fullest. It is our hope that our Diet for Life will do the same for you.

PART ONE

Coming Back from Near Death to Glowing Health and Vitality: Our Story

1

The End:
It Was the Beginning
of Our New Life

The day the cardiologist told my husband he was going to die, my world came to an end. Yet, looking back, it was the day our whole new world was born.

Our story begins about two months before that day.

The Attacks

That spring night in 1974 started, much like any other of our Saturday nights in those days, with an elegant meal at home for just the two of us. I was always planning gastronomic delights for Harold, and that night my *pièce de résistance* was the classic Steak Diane, my style. "A masterpiece," Harold called it. It was accompanied by *pommes frites* and sautéed *haricots verts*. It was preceded by cocktails, hors d'oeuvres, and a mixed green salad with my own flavorful dressing; and followed with a *baba au rhum* topped with *crème Chantilly*. Harold had discovered an exquisite Cabernet Sauvignon from a small California vineyard, and it had been a perfect companion for the steak.

After dinner, we settled down in front of the TV for an evening of basketball. Harold had been an avid basketball fan since his college days. That night the New York Knicks were playing. It was a close, exciting game. The outcome wasn't decided until the final seconds. Harold yelled, applauded, leaped to his feet, and, when the Knicks lost, groaned.

One room in our Manhattan apartment is Harold's workshop. He went into it and closed the door. I thought he would sulk for a few minutes—what ardent fan doesn't after a loss?—then come out and, with a smile on his face, say, "Well, you can't win 'em all." It was a ritual we went through. But minutes passed and the door stayed closed. My woman's instincts are strong—I can trust them—and I knew he wasn't brooding about the lost game. Something was wrong.

I knocked on the door.

"Are you all right?"

No answer.

"Harold! Are you all right?"

I heard strange sounds, as if he were choking.

Then he said, "I'm okay. I'll be out soon."

I went back to the living room. But he didn't come out soon. I knocked on the door again.

He came out holding his chest. He went straight to the bathroom. I could hear him throwing up.

He came out after a long time and said, "Look, I've had too much rich food, too much excitement, so my stomach's upset, and I'm going to be running to the bathroom all night. I don't want to disturb you, so I'll sleep on the couch in my workshop tonight, okay?"

"Okay."

But my instincts told me it wasn't.

Neither of us open a closed door without knocking. But later that night I did. He was lying on the couch, sweating profusely, clutching his chest. His face was shiny and red. He was making those strange choking sounds. I was frightened.

"I'm going to call a doctor," I said.

"For an upset stomach? Ridiculous! Look, here's a prediction: I'll be right as rain in the morning. Now let's both get some sleep."

I couldn't. I looked in on him often during the night. He was sleeping peacefully. In the morning, he was fine.

"Told you so," he said.

I was glad he had been right. But I was still worried.

That day, Sunday, we had a sausage-and-egg brunch, read *The New York Times* together, listened to some Beethoven and Lerner and Loewe on the stereo, and soaked up rest. We had a dinner engagement with another couple. Harold slipped into a new custom-made blazer, and he looked splendid. Our friends called for us at our apartment. We had a round of drinks, then walked to a new Italian restaurant highly praised by New York's leading food critic.

It was a smallish place, overcrowded and hot. The service was frenetic. The food was greasy and heavily salted. I felt sick to my stomach after only sampling the meal. But Harold ate everything on his plate with gusto.

At 9:30 that night, back in our apartment, the symptoms of the previous night returned. But they were far worse than before. He threw up frequently. He clutched at his chest, then, as the night wore on, at his arms, at the back of his neck, at his chin. He was drenched in perspiration. There was a terrifying new symptom, too. He was bringing up gas continually and painfully.

I tried to get my internist. The answering service said he would call back. I called again and again, but he never called back.

When Harold awoke on Monday morning, I could see he was still in pain. I called my internist, and this time I was able to get through. I described the symptoms. He recommended a cardiologist. I called him, told him what had happened. He said, "Come right over."

I said to Harold, "Get dressed. We're going to see a doctor. He's expecting us."

He began to get dressed.

That shook me up more than my internist telling me to see a cardiologist. Harold had never seen a doctor in the thirteen years we had known each other. It was a matter of pride to handle his illnesses himself. If Harold agreed to see a doctor, he must be very sick.

The cardiologist took an electrocardiogram (E.K.G.). It's a record of the electrical activity produced by the heart as it contracts and relaxes. It looks like the zigzag lines on a graph. By examining it, a cardiologist can tell whether the heart is functioning normally or whether it has been damaged.

The cardiologist looked at Harold's E.K.G. and said, "Mr. Prince, you may have had a heart attack. Then again, you may not."

I wanted to know what happened last night and the night before.

He shrugged. "Maybe he had a heart attack on one of those nights, or on both of those nights, or on none of those nights."

"What should we do now?"

"Nothing. Just take it easy."

On the way home in the cab, Harold and I stared at each other in disbelief. The cardiologist didn't know what had happened. Worse: Harold was very sick, and he offered no help.

"Let's say it amounts to this," Harold said. "I didn't have a heart attack, and everything's going to be all right."

But my instincts told me differently. They were right.

Three hours after we were back in the apartment, another attack hit him. It was far worse than the preceding two. He was in excruciating pain. I thought he was going to die.

I called the cardiologist. He arranged for immediate hospitalization.

The next few months would be the most miserable of our lives.

The Hospital

The intensive-care unit was like a science-fiction setting. White dominated. White shiny walls. White masks. White uniforms. White tables and chairs. The white was broken only by the grays, blacks, and silvers of medical instruments, and the pale green faces of the electronic monitors to which Harold was connected by wires. From a transparent container hung on a pole, glucose dripped through a rubber tube into his artery. The monitors emitted electronic beeps.

Three doctors surrounded his bed. They machinegunned commands and questions at him.

"Don't ask questions, just answer them. . . ."

"Lie down. Breathe in. Breath out. Again."

"How old are you?"

"When did you first get the symptoms?"

"What were the symptoms?"

"Describe the pain."

"We don't want your opinion. Just give us the facts."

I said, "Did he have a heart attack?"

One doctor said to me, "Don't interrupt."

Another doctor said to me, "Wait outside, Mrs. Prince."

I went into the corridor and stood by the closed door of the intensive-care unit. I wondered why our cardiologist wasn't with Harold. Then I began to think about Harold's family. One of his brothers had died of a heart attack. Another had had two heart attacks and several strokes. His father had died of a heart attack when he was about Harold's age.

The door opened sharply. One of the doctors stood in the doorway and said, "Here are his clothes. He won't need them."

Slam went the door.

I carried his clothes out of the hospital, my eyes welling up with tears. Somewhere on the street I found a torn shopping bag. I placed his clothes in it, then walked the three blocks back to our apartment in a daze. I still didn't know if he had had a heart attack. Why didn't they tell me what was happening?

When I visited Harold the following day, the cardiologist was at his bedside. The doctor was brusque.

"His condition seems to be stable," he said to me. "Many tests have to be taken." Exit.

The next day when I visited Harold, he glared at me. When I caressed his cheek, he shoved my hand away. He looked as if he hated me. It was a terrifying reversal of personality.

I phoned the cardiologist.

"He's just depressed," he said. "It's natural. People get depressed when they have a heart attack."

That's how I learned Harold had had a heart attack.

But it didn't explain his personality change. I had seen Harold depressed before. But even at his lowest ebb, he had never shown anything but love and kindness toward me. I was sure the drugs they were giving him were responsible for the sudden change. I was right.

Harold had never taken a drug in all our years together, not even an aspirin. Now they were dosing him with Valium during the day and Dalmane at night. Valium calms down some people, agitates others, and depresses still others. A doctor never knows in advance what it will do. It depressed Harold. Dalmane is a sleeping pill which can produce a depressive hangover. The two pills working together had turned Harold into a man I didn't know.

The cardiologist refused to take him off the drugs. "It's only natural he should feel upset and not sleep well in a hospital," he told me. "The drugs will calm him down and give him a good night's sleep."

Wouldn't friendly care, smiling faces, a congenial atmosphere, and an honest talk with Harold about his condition and what was being done to help him be more effective than tranquilizers? The cardiologist didn't answer me.

The next day when I entered Harold's room, there was no one in it. I was frantic until I discovered that he had been transferred to another intensive-care unit. This was a small narrow room in which three beds, placed only a few feet apart, were occupied by cardiac patients. Over each bed a TV set was suspended from the ceiling. Visitors were permitted from early morning to late night. There was a constant din from voices, the TV sets, and the beeps and bells of the monitoring devices. It was a nerve-wracking place even for somebody in perfect health.

Was this the way to treat a man who just had had a heart attack? I received no answer from the cardiologist.

After three days in that room, Harold was removed from intensive care. He was wheel-chaired to a semi-private room. His roommate had a disease which was treated by painting a large part of his body each day with iodine. The stench was unbearable. The first time I visited Harold in that room I nearly gagged. And Harold was supposed to live, eat, and sleep in that room.

"No way," I told the head nurse. "I want him out of there."

"Instead of complaining," she snapped at me, "why don't you feel sorry for that poor man in the room with your husband? Remember, he has rights, too."

What about my husband? He was paying $275 a day for his room. Didn't he at least have the right to a clean-smelling place in which to recuperate? The cardiologist told me there was nothing he could do. For the rest of his stay in the hospital, Harold spent most of his waking hours sitting on a bench in the corridor.

The cardiologist visited Harold there every day except on weekends. The routine never varied. The cardiologist would ask Harold how he felt, Harold would answer "Okay," and the cardiologist would depart. Later, when the cardiologist's bill arrived, we found each "How do you feel?" cost $50.

The only place they would serve Harold food was in his room, but the stench there killed his appetite. Even under the best conditions, Harold would have had difficulty forcing the food down. It was overcooked, swimming in grease, heavily salted. Harold ate very little, and he was growing weaker.

The stress of hospital life, the drugs, the long days in the corridor, and the lack of food were doing terrible things to him. On his seventeenth day in the hospital, he was so weak he could hardly stand. He was flatulent. He ran his hand frequently over his forehead, as if to rub away pain. There was no color in his cheeks, no glimmer of light in his eyes, no smile ever. He didn't answer when I spoke to him. His attitude toward me was hostile. He had become a stranger—a frightening stranger. He was, in many ways, far worse than when he was admitted.

The cardiologist called me. He said I could take Harold home.

We left the hospital with prescriptions for three drugs in addition to the Valium and Dalmane: Nitroglycerine to treat chest pains (angina pectoris); Hydrodiuril to reduce high blood pressure; and Inderal to slow the rate of Harold's heartbeat (on the theory that the slower the heartbeat, the less the chance of a heart attack). The five drugs in concert made Harold sluggish, stupid, and headachy. They merely added to his hostility and depression. They did nothing to alleviate his chest pains and flatulence.

I called the cardiologist and pleaded with him to do something.

"Let's see how bad he really is," he said. "I want him to take a stress test. Then we'll see what can be done."

The Test

The idea behind the stress test is this:

When you walk fast or climb a hill, you're under stress. When you're under stress, your heart needs more blood. The heart draws in this blood by a pumping action—a heartbeat. If there's a normal amount of blood in the arteries leading to the heart, a certain number of pumping actions—heartbeats—per minute are needed to provide the required blood. If there's less than a normal amount of blood in those arteries, more pumping actions—more heartbeats—per minute are needed to bring in the same amount of blood. There's less blood in the arteries when they're clogged. So if your heart beats faster than it normally should under stress, that's evidence that your arteries are clogged.

Harold's stress test was conducted by a private testing company recommended by the cardiologist. A nurse and a doctor were in attendance as Harold, in shorts and sneakers and hooked up by wires to a monitoring device, stepped on a treadmill. The nurse pushed a button, and the treadmill began to move progressively faster. At the same time, it gradually tilted upward. It seemed to Harold as if he were walking more and more rapidly up an increasingly steep slope. The monitoring device electronically recorded the number of his heartbeats per minute.

A printout from the monitor was sent to the cardiologist. From it he could not only tell if there was blockage, but also what arteries were affected, and to what extent they were clogged. He held the printout in his hands as we sat in front of his desk in his office.

"Mr. Prince," he said, "your heart's getting very little blood. All three major arteries to your heart are clogged. If you walk just one city block vigorously, you'll drop dead."

That was how he told me my husband was going to die.

"There's only one chance," he said. "Bypass surgery. There's no time to lose. I'll call the hospital and arrange for the angiogram right now."

He reached for the phone.

"Hold it," Harold said. "I want to think this over."

The Decision

On the way back home in the cab, Harold explained that there was something in his head about the surgery, about something else, but he couldn't think about anything clearly because of the drugs. When we returned to the apartment, he took the containers of Valium and Dalmane from his medicine chest and threw them in the garbage.

"Look," he said, "for myself, I don't care whether I live or die. But I can't leave you alone. In a few days my brain will be clear, and we'll talk."

For the next three days he suffered withdrawal symptoms: nausea, dizziness, a feeling of malaise. On the fourth day after breakfast he said he was ready to talk.

He said the angiogram is dangerous. I knew that. It's accomplished by inserting a tube into the arm or groin, and then snaking it up an artery toward the heart. It takes hours and is performed without anesthesia. The slightest slip could be fatal. Dye is pumped through the tube into the artery. When the dye is in the artery, there's less room for oxygen. When a heart is starved of oxygen, it stops. It's happened.

The dye is necessary to make a clear X-ray picture of the artery leading to the heart—the angiogram. Using it as a guide, the surgeon locates the area of maximum blockage. He snips a piece of clean vein from the leg or mammary gland, and attaches one end to the artery just in front of the area of maximum blockage, and the other end to the artery just behind it. There's now a loop around that area. The blood passes through it, bypassing the blockage. Since angina and heart attack are caused by an insufficient flow of blood reaching the heart, bypass surgery was hailed as a miracle cure for both maladies.

I knew it really wasn't. Although it cured angina in many cases, it failed in some. A woman I knew underwent two bypass operations and came out of them with worse angina each time. There was also no evidence that it prolonged life. One of Harold's dearest friends was cured of angina by a bypass, but died of a heart attack within a year.

"And it's extremely dangerous," Harold said. "The odds are only one out of ten that I'll survive the operation. I can get better odds as a combat soldier in Vietnam."

He pointed out our health insurance benefits were almost gone, the operation would cost thousands, it would keep him away from work for months, and it would leave us destitute. "Besides," he added, "nothing will drag me back into that hospital again."

"But if you don't agree to the operation, what chance will you have?" I asked.

"A good one," he said. "I got the idea in a sort of a flash the moment the cardiologist said I was just as good as dead. Now I've thought it out, and I know there's another way."

"What kind of way?"

"A diet," he said.

It was to develop into our Diet for Life.

2

The Diet for Life Is Born

The Diet for Life did not spring into existence overnight. There was a long, hard struggle ahead of me. The basic diet Harold had chosen was virtually inedible. There would be months of misery while we tried to cope with it. There would be a time of despair when it seemed Harold could no longer stay on it.

But the life of the man I loved was at stake, and that gave me the strength to do what others said was impossible—transform the basic diet, made up almost entirely of unappetizing foods, into the new haute cuisine of health. Ask Harold today what the essential ingredient of the Diet for Life is, and he'll answer: Love.

But for the first several months, my hands were tied.

The Restrictions

In the '60s Harold had ghosted a best-selling book on heart attack (it sold more than 250,000 copies in hardcover alone). It was the first book to take a nutritional approach to the prevention and cure of cardiac diseases. From his work on that book, Harold knew he would have to lose weight, and he would have to reduce sharply his intake of two nutrients indicated by scientific researchers as contributing to artery blockage: fats, particularly saturated fats, and cholesterol.

The book recommended a diet designed to do just that. It was invented by Dr. Norman Jolliffe, and it also eliminated the use of sugar (sucrose). Harold and I examined other diets, and we concluded Dr. Jolliffe's Prudent Diet was the one for us (the story is in the next chapter). At once we cut down on fats/saturated fats, cholesterol, and sugar.

But Dr. Jolliffe's diet was invented in the early '60s. This was 1974—and what had science discovered since then?

Both of us had kept up in a general way with advances in nutrition, but we now engaged in an in-depth study of the scientific literature. We found that in those 14 years much progress had been made by scientific researchers (not practicing physicians) in relating faulty nutrition not only to heart attack, but to all degenerative diseases. These include high blood pressure (hypertension), diabetes, hypoglycemia (low blood sugar), gout, and stroke. There was also much hardcore data on sound nutrition as a means of reaching peak health both mentally and physically, and staying there for the rest of your life.

We received help from Harold's son Barry. He had given up a successful career as a motion-picture writer-director to study nutrition. Now phone calls from Woodacre, California, where he made his home, brought us a constant stream of up-to-date nutritional information.

When we analyzed all the material we had gathered, we discovered that Dr. Jolliffe's restrictions were just the tip of the iceberg. We would also have to eliminate salt, pepper (white and black), caffeine, alcohol, artificial sweeteners, and chemical additives. In addition, all *varieties* of sugar and salt were prohibited: confectioner's sugar, turbinado sugar, brown sugar, raw sugar, molasses, corn and maple syrup; sea salt, kosher salt, and seaweed preparations like kelp and dulse.

No food containing any restricted ingredient was acceptable. As I wheeled my shopping cart past each category of food in the supermarket, DON'T EAT signs flashed in my brain. (In the following list of DON'T EATs, the categories are arranged alphabetically.)

BREADS AND ROLLS:

DON'T EAT: all, including melba toast, zwieback, Swedish flatbreads, saltsticks, pita and dietetic breads. (Baking powder and baking soda were also forbidden.)

CONDIMENTS, SAUCES, AND SALAD DRESSINGS:

DON'T EAT: ketchup, chutney and other relishes, all prepared mustards (except low-sodium), tabasco, all bottled sauces including soy and other Oriental sauces, monosodium glutamate (M.S.G.), dietetic and all other salad dressings.

DAIRY PRODUCTS:

DON'T EAT: butter, whole milk, most cheeses, sweet or sour cream, whole-milk yogurt, low-fat yogurt with fruit flavorings, synthetic dessert whips, coffee whiteners, and egg yolks.

DELICATESSEN:

DON'T EAT: corned beef, pastrami, sausages, liverwurst and other wursts, pâtés and spreads, bologna, salami, frankfurters, and luncheon meats; potato salad, cole slaw, vegetable salads, meat and fish salads, olives, sauerkraut, pickles, pickled onions, and other pickled vegetables; ethnic specialties.

DESSERTS:

DON'T EAT: ice cream, ice milk, sherbets, ices, mousses, custards, puddings, flavored gelatin, fruit toppings, syrups, candy, chocolate, pies, pastries, cakes, crackers, cookies, jellies, jams, preserves, and most nut spreads.

FATS AND OILS:

DON'T EAT: lard and other animal fats, hardened white vegetable shortenings (hydrogenated vegetable fats), most margarines, mayonnaise, butter, and other fatty dairy products; palm and coconut oil, and peanut and olive oil (except in limited quantities).

FISH AND SHELLFISH:

DON'T EAT: lobster, crayfish, mussels, clams, scallops, octopus, squid, shrimp (except in small quantities), and fatty fish like rainbow trout; caviar and other fish roe; smoked and/or salted fish; most canned and frozen fish.

FRUITS AND VEGETABLES:

DON'T EAT: Canned fruit in light or heavy syrup, frozen fruit with sugar added, almost all canned vegetables, frozen vegetables with salt added; coconuts and avocados; sweetened juices.

GOURMET FOODS:

DON'T EAT: all, with a few exceptions including a salt-free Dijon mustard, and canned chestnuts, water chestnuts, and horseradish paste or powder, none of which contains added salt.

MEATS AND POULTRY:

DON'T EAT: fatty cuts of meat (most prime cuts), tongue, kidneys, brains, sweetbreads, liver (except in small amounts), lungs, tripe, bacon and other salted and/or smoked meats, canned meats, duck, capon, roaster chickens, and goose.

PREPARED FOODS:

DON'T EAT: all commercially prepared foods, including frozen baked goods, frozen meals, and TV dinners.

SNACKS:

DON'T EAT: all commercial snacks, including potato chips, cheese puffs, popcorn, pretzels, and dips and spreads; almost all nuts.

SOUPS:

DON'T EAT: all canned soups, dried soup mixes, and bouillon cubes.

And as I passed by beverages in the supermarket or in the window of my favorite liquor store, a DON'T DRINK sign lit up in my mind.

BEVERAGES:

DON'T DRINK: coffee, tea, most herb teas, milk drinks, thick shakes, chocolate drinks, cocoa, all soft drinks, distilled water, and all mineral waters (except those labeled low in sodium); all beers, ales, malt liquors, hard liquors, wines, and liqueurs.

The DON'T EAT and DON'T DRINK signs went on as well when I passed take-out places, and all restaurants including health-food restaurants.

There was little enjoyable food left to eat. To make matters worse, Harold imposed these additional dietary limitations on me:

- *Meat twice a week.* We had been eating meat daily, sometimes three times a day. We had been eating tender, prime cuts. Now we were to eat lean and less tender choice cuts.
- *Chicken twice a week.* We had eaten chicken occasionally, and then only fatty roasters. (We preferred capon, goose, and duck.) Now we were to eat broilers, which are less fatty and less tasty; and the skin, which gives them much of their taste, had to be removed before cooking. I had never done that before.

- *Fish twice a week.* And Harold abhorred fish. He would eat it only in restaurants where it was broiled under extremely high heat to drive off the fishy taste and odor. Neither my broiler nor oven could supply that kind of heat.
- *At all other times—fruits, vegetables, and grains.* Harold loathed vegetarian meals.
- *And I was to use no marinades, seasonings, or flavorings whatsoever.* Many nutrition experts had concluded that plain food is healthy food; and although there was no scientific basis for their judgment, Harold decided to take no chances and go along with it.

The meals were awful.

"Look," Harold said after a while, "I've got to stay with it, but you don't. Make my food for me, and make your food for you. Okay?"

"Okay."

But that was worse. Preparing separate meals for each of us meant more than twice as much work. But I could have put up with that. What I couldn't cope with was the sense of separation that I felt each time we sat down at the table. Sharing food with someone you love is one of the most intimate and rewarding of life's experiences, but now at every meal I felt we were miles apart. I soon stopped making one dish for him and another dish for me. Harold's diet became my diet.

I hated it. We couldn't even escape to a restaurant once in a while. There was no relief from the round of dull-to-repugnant breakfasts, lunches, and dinners. But as long as it was helping Harold, I'd grin and bear it. But after about three months, I knew it wasn't helping him. It was harming him.

He had set out to lose about 15 pounds, and he had done it; but he continued to lose weight. He looked poorly. His complexion was sallow. There was none of his old flashing wit. He was dull. He lacked energy. He was letting his assignments slide. A book he was writing under contract was long overdue.

What disturbed me most was that his cardiac symptoms seemed to grow worse. He clutched his chest frequently. His painful flatulence increased. I would wake up at night to see if he was breathing. Every time he went out for a walk, my heart wouldn't stop pounding until he returned.

I could see he hated the diet even more than I did. He would take a bite of a dinner dish and say, "I'm not hungry. Let's save it. I'll have it for lunch tomorrow." He never did. He ate less and less. I knew it was only a matter of time before he went off the diet. And if he did, then there would be no hope except bypass surgery—and that could kill him, but there was no evidence that it could cure him.

I was in a state of despair. I had to do something. I tossed the problem around in my mind. The diet was nutritionally sound, but something had gone wrong. Why? I had my own theory. No matter how nutritionally valuable a diet is, if you don't enjoy what you're eating, it's no good for you. Healthful food prepared distastefully is unhealthful food. I thought: If I could prepare healthful foods tastefully—more than tastefully—excitingly, deliciously, then Harold would eat with joy again, and the diet would have a chance to work.

I told Harold I would like to try to make the food tastier. Would he allow me to use marinades, seasonings, and flavorings? He agreed ("Anything would be better than what we're eating") with the proviso that I stick to our basic meal plan, and use only healthful ingredients—no DON'T EAT's and DON'T DRINK's.

Perhaps diet cookbooks could guide me. I bought all I could lay my hands on. Some eliminated salt, but were high in fats, cholesterol, and sugar. Others were low in fats and cholesterol, but were high in sugar and salt. Sugar-free cookbooks were high in salt, cholesterol, and fats. No single cookbook was low in fats/saturated fats, cholesterol, and used no sugar or salt. And all diet cookbooks were packed with our DON'T EAT's and DON'T DRINK's. I tried to adapt some of the more promising recipes to our diet, but they had been concocted by clinicians, not chefs, and the dishes tasted like something synthesized in a laboratory. Dead end.

I was on my own. Starting from scratch, I would have to create a new cuisine based on healthful ingredients—a cuisine that would be varied, innovative, and delectable. "Impossible!" my friends and relatives said. They reflected the opinions of the nation's leading food critics who held that no healthful food could be made even palatable. (Since then one of the most eminent of those critics has come down with a degenerative disease, and has followed the lead of *The Dieter's Gourmet Cookbook* with a restricted-diet cookbook of his own, albeit one still high in forbidden ingredients.)

But I didn't care who said it was impossible. I was determined to succeed. I had to bring my husband back to the joys of the dining table to keep him from the dangers of the operating table.

The Breakthroughs

I started with enormous advantages. I had been cooking ever since I was a child, and I'm very good at it. I had been trained in classic French cuisine. During numerous trips to Europe with Harold, I had studied the dishes of many nations (the *brio* of Italian cookery continues to fascinate me). In my apartment, one of this nation's leading Chinese chefs had taught me the secrets of his country's culinary arts. I had taught myself how to reproduce the exotic masterpieces of India and the Near East. I could begin to create my new haute cuisine of health backed up by my talent in the kitchen, nearly a lifetime of experience, and my knowledge of the great cooking styles of the world.

I began with an exciting new premise. All the diet recipes I had read were based on the premise that the taste of your favorite dishes would not be altered substantially by eliminating forbidden ingredients (say, salt), or substituting for forbidden ingredients (say, sorbitol for sugar), or cutting down on the quantities of forbidden ingredients (say, one egg yolk instead of two). It was a premise that never worked. Take salt out of familiar dishes, for example, and what's left is dull, flat, and insipid. My new premise was this: that using only healthful ingredients, original dishes could be created with new stimulating flavors, and with basic qualities everybody looks for in some of their foods: sweetness, creaminess, the taste of fat, and texture.

My first task was to find the healthful ingredients which could do all this. That meant more research. I studied government publications on nutrition, food-company literature, shelves of books on foodstuffs. I read everything on labels in supermarkets and health-food stores (and came up with a shocker: not everything in health-food stores is healthful). I spent long hours experimenting in my kitchen. I had to work fast—I couldn't rid myself of the feeling that time was quickly running out for Harold—and in a short time I came up with a list of healthful ingredients with which I could make my premise work.

Here's a tip-of-the-iceberg view of that list. (The ingredients are discussed in some detail throughout the book. The subject index will guide you to them.)

For new stimulating tastes I relied heavily on herbs and spices. I cooked with them; I sprinkled them on foods. Fresh herbs are utterly delicious, but only a few of them—dill, parsley, basil, tarragon, garlic, and shallots—were easily obtainable then in New York. All the other herbs I used were dried, but by combining them in the right amounts (long, long hours of trial and error), I came up with wonderful new taste sensations. (Books on the use of herbs were so general in their instructions that they were of virtually no help to me.) Garlic or shallots alone made salt superfluous.

For sweetness in desserts and cooked foods—and even in breads—I used fresh and cooked fruits, fresh fruit juices, and bottled fruit juices without added sugar, as well as sweet herbs and spices, including allspice, anise, cinnamon, coriander, ginger, mace, nutmeg, sweet basil, and tarragon. In some dishes I included sweet vegetables like carrots, tomatoes, and onions. Date powder (which I found in health-food stores) earned a place among my favored sweeteners, as did honey, which I used sparingly. (Honey is not potentially harmful sucrose, but a mixture of glucose and fructose.)

For creaminess I settled on one brand of dry non-fat milk (after experimenting with every brand on the market) which is so sweet and rich that it proved to be the answer to "How can you make a creamy sauce without cream?" To make it taste even better, I prepared it with spring water low in sodium.

For the taste of fat I selected corn oil after trying all high-polyunsaturated oils available in supermarkets, health-food stores, and gourmet shops. By far the tastiest of all healthful oils, it is equally wonderful in cooked foods, salad dressings, and in my mayonnaise-type spread (the recipe for which you'll find in *The Dieter's Gourmet Cookbook*). It mixes heavenly with small quantities of olive oil. Fat tastes came, too, from several low-fat cheeses which I used in soups and sandwiches, and in dips and salads.

For texture, corn oil provided crispness to sautéed dishes, moistness to baked products, and smoothness to salad dressings. Some vegetables and high-polyunsaturated nuts imparted crunchiness to a variety of dishes. Egg whites gave a fine texture to baked goods and omelettes (made without egg yolks!). And my innovative marinades tenderized choice cuts of meats and broiler chickens (and also helped to enhance the flavor of fish).

Dish by dish, my new haute cuisine of health was taking shape. But one problem remained, and it was a formidable one: bread. Harold had outlawed all commercial breads, even the dietetic varieties; and bread deprivation was far more painful to him than dessert deprivation (it is to many dieters). My problem was to make breads without salt, sugar, fats, or cholesterol—and to make them full-textured, crusty, and delicious.

I solved the problem in three ways. I used various combinations (determined experimentally) of rye, buckwheat, whole wheat, gluten, and unbleached flours. I added sweet spices and herbs, unsweetened fruit juices, and mixtures of seeds. I developed new techniques for making delectable loaves in an ordinary apartment oven.

Low in calories, my breads—and I created a dozen or so varieties—were a delight on our table. So were my rolls. I even made my own bread crumbs for breadings and stuffings. Years later a leading food critic would call my bread and rolls, made only with healthful ingredients, "better than any kind of bread you can buy in a store." (Bread recipes begin on page 189.)

Six months had passed, and Harold seemed to be doing well on my new cuisine. He was looking better. His color had improved. He was more energetic. In good weather, he walked a mile each day. The angina had abated somewhat, and his bouts of painful flatulence occurred less frequently.

He stopped using Hydrodiuril when he began to reduce (I'll tell you why in the next chapter), and he was on only two drugs, Nitroglycerine and Inderal. The Nitroglycerine gave him headaches, and the Inderal slowed down his thinking, but he was back at work, and his attitude toward me had ceased to be hostile. He was far from his old self, still withdrawn and gloomy, but he had begun to communicate again, and that was a good sign.

One afternoon he said to me, "What're we having for dinner tonight?"

I smiled. "If it's Tuesday," I said, "it must be chicken. But tonight," I added, "it's a premiere—sautéed chicken with pimentos."

He went out for a walk, then returned with a familiar-shaped package under his arm—a shape I hadn't seen in our home in almost a year.

He unwrapped it and said, "In honor of chicken with pimentos—and all the other great dishes you've created to make my life beautiful again—I've bought this elegant wine to drink a toast to you."

I was elated.

I bought fresh flowers, and set the dinner table with more than usual care. I created a new rice dish, my version of an Italian risotto, to accompany the chicken with pimentos. The salad would be a first, too: arrugula and endive with a dressing he had never tasted before. And for dessert I whipped up another innovation: a pineapple sherbet (which years later a prominent food critic would hail as "outshining ice cream.") Calorie count, including wine, was less than 840 (similar dishes made with DON'T EAT's would have contributed 3,000 calories or more).

My food was a smash success. The wine was a dream. (Over the dinner table Harold told me that new research had revealed that wine in moderate amounts was not harmful and that it actually helped prevent heart attack. So wine was off our no-no list. We could drink it, and I could cook with it—and that was wonderful news.) For the first time since he had entered the hospital, we smiled at each other, touched, kissed. We were together again.

I had made many breakthroughs in the previous six months, but this was the biggest breakthrough of them all. I was so happy I don't remember crying.

The Victory

I had found the key to Harold's recovery, and nothing could stop me now. My mind was always on another new recipe, another new technique, another new flavor—another new surprise for Harold. I would even awake in the middle of the night with new ideas dancing in my head, and hurry to jot them down before they vanished like a dream.

The exciting food lifted his spirits, and that lifted mine. He had added vitamin supplements to his diet, and his recovery was steady now. There was little angina; painful flatulence was rare. In another year, there was no flatulence at all; the angina was only a memory. He threw away his Nitroglycerine and his Inderal. He's not taken another drug since.

My new haute cuisine of health, plus vitamin supplements, became our Diet for Life. After three years on it, my husband, who had been told by a cardiologist he would drop dead if he walked one city block vigorously, climbed a mountain. You should see him now, seven years after his heart attack—slender, beautifully complexioned, full of vigor. He's 65 but looks at least 10 years younger. His general health is superb.

So is his sexual prowess. Ours had been a mad, mad love affair; and up until his heart attack, sex had been one of the peak experiences of our lives. There were two lonely, frustrating years when we were too frightened to have intercourse. But now our sex life is more beautiful than it's ever been. (The story is in Chapter 14.)

His energy level in all phases of life is unbelievable. He's writing four books concurrently, works 12 hours a day, often seven days a week. His latest book—a fascinating review for laymen of the great discoveries in five branches of modern science—has been greeted with rave reviews. It's the selection of two book clubs, and has been translated into Italian, Dutch, and Japanese.

He's a new man emotionally, too. Before his heart attack, he had been more interested in ideas than in people. But now he likes to be with people, can empathize with them. He's outgoing, convivial, self-assured. He's a happy man.

And I'm a happy woman.

It was a great victory which Harold and I share. But, looking back, the basic recipe was simple: To healthful foods, add great dollops of love. Continuously.

That victory which we won for ourselves, we're passing on to you with our Diet for Life.

PART TWO

The Diet for Life Eating Plan for Healthfully Slimming Down to Ideal Weight— and Staying There for the Rest of Your Life

3

An Analysis of Popular Diets— from the Deadly to the Prudent

When Harold was in his early 30s—and that was many years before I met him—he tells me he was a fat man. (It's so hard to believe.) He weighed 180 pounds on a five-foot, two-inch frame. He decided to reduce, and his family doctor prescribed a diet. It was stunningly effective. In one summer he lost 50 pounds. His waist shrank from 46 to 32, his collar size from 16½ to 14½, his suit size from 44 extra-stout to 36 short. When he dropped weight, he told me, he dropped years in looks and gained energy and self-assurance.

But 25 years later, he was to place much of the blame for his heart attack on that very diet.

The Deadly Doctor's Diet

What his doctor had prescribed for him was a variation of the then-popular high-protein diet. The daily menus followed this basic pattern:

> *Breakfast.* One-half grapefruit. Two boiled eggs. Black coffee or tea sweetened with saccharin.
> *Lunch.* A quarter-pound of cold cuts. One slice of bread. Coffee or tea sweetened with saccharin.
> *Dinner.* A quarter-pound of meat (steak, chops, and roast beef preferred). Small portions of low-carbohydrate vegetables like asparagus and cabbage. Saccharin-sweetened gelatin dessert. Coffee or tea sweetened with saccharin.
> *At all meals.* All the condiments, relishes, pickles, and bottled sauces he could eat.

The diet contributed about 1,200 calories a day. Of those calories, 7.5 percent came from carbohydrates, 33 percent from proteins, and a whopping 59.5 percent from fats. (The percentages of these nutrients are expressed here, as they are throughout this book, in terms of total daily caloric intake.) The doctor's diet, like most so-called high-protein diets in those days (the early 1950s), was not a high-protein diet at all, but a high-fat diet. It was high, as well, in saturated fat, cholesterol, and salt.

It was a diet that, working slowly over the years, could bring on high blood pressure, atherosclerosis (artery blockage), and subsequent heart attack. Upping calories to maintain weight, Harold stayed on a gourmet version of this meat-oriented, fat-rich diet (he never ate potatoes; always limited himself to one slice of bread a day) until all three degenerative diseases struck.

When, after his heart attack, Harold returned from the hospital, he weighed 125 pounds, the average weight for a small-boned American male his size. But, examining the most recent studies of body weight as it related to health, we were shocked to discover he was overweight. Statistical studies made by insurance companies showed that there was an ideal weight at which Americans of a certain height would be likely to live long and healthy lives. Harold's ideal weight is 110. That meant he had to lose 15 pounds. (You'll find a chart of ideal weights on page 59. They're considerably lower than average weights, proof that the average American is more than moderately overweight.)

The problem we faced was this: How was he to lose those 15 pounds? We discovered that in addition to Dr. Jolliffe's Prudent Diet, we had three popular kinds of diets to choose from: a true high-protein diet, a high-fat diet, and a high-carbohydrate diet. We investigated each before we decided the best way to lose weight was on Harold's stringent modification of Dr. Jolliffe's Diet. (It was unpleasant. But transformed by my new haute cuisine of health, that diet is now a delicious and joyful way to reduce without any sense of deprivation.)

We set up this test for each diet:

	NO	MAYBE	YES
DOES IT WORK?	☐	☐	☐
IS IT HEALTHFUL?	☐	☐	☐
CAN YOU STAY ON IT?	☐	☐	☐

This is the result of our investigations in terms of the current prime example of each kind of diet: the Tarnower (Scarsdale) Diet, a high-protein diet; the Atkins Diet, a high-fat diet; the Pritikin Diet, a high-carbohydrate diet; and the Diet for Life, a modified Prudent Diet.

What's Wrong with the Tarnower Diet?

The late Dr. Herman Tarnower reported that his diet averages 43 percent protein, 22.5 percent fat, 34.5 percent carbohydrates, and 1,000 calories or less per day.

Does it work? If you're eager to shed poundage rapidly, a diet of this kind has an irresistible appeal—you can lose up to five to six pounds a week for the first two weeks. It works so well during this period not because it's a high-protein diet, but because it's a low-carbohydrate diet. Its carbohydrate content is a stunning 23.5 percentage points lower than the percentage recommended by the Federal Dietary Guidelines. Here's what happens:

Carbohydrates cling to water. When carbohydrate intake is reduced, some water is freed and flushed out of the body through the kidneys. Water is heavy—a pint weighs a pound. On the Tarnower Diet, three to four pounds of water can be flushed away in the first two weeks—and that's the major source of the amazing weight loss. (Additional weight is lost due to lowered calorie intake.)

After the first two weeks most of the carbohydrate-held water has been released, and further weight reduction depends on restricting yourself to 1,000 calories a day or less. For the average American weight is now shed at about two pounds a week, which is a sensible rate of weight loss.

No question—you *can* lose weight on the Tarnower Diet.

Is it healthful? The Tarnower Diet's 1,000 calories a day or less (an independent analysis sets the figure at 887) is below the safety limit of 1,200 set by the Federal Dietary Guidelines. Below that limit there is a possibility of vitamin and mineral deficiencies. Tarnower contends, however, that "you won't develop any vitamin deficiency in two weeks, even on a starvation diet," so no vitamin or mineral supplements are prescribed.

But the major potential hazard from this diet arises from its high protein content. The National Academy of Science's National Research Council has specified a Recommended Daily Allowance (R.D.A.) of 56 grams of protein for the average male and 46 grams for the average female. On the Tarnower Diet, the daily allowance is about 107 grams. (It's about 111 grams on the Weight Watcher's Diet, another high-protein diet.) What are some possible effects?

- Excess protein can speed up the body's engine when there's no need for it (like idling the motor of your car). This can shorten the lives of some cells, and bring on symptoms of premature aging.
- The amount of uric acid—one of the breakdown products of protein—can rise markedly in the bloodstream. Uric acid forms as tiny crystals, and excess amounts can deposit in the joints, causing the excruciating pain of gout, a disease once prevalent among the British aristocracy who subsisted mainly on meat.

• Excess uric acid is also a poison. When it is not washed out of the body in the urine (as in the case of kidney malfunction), its accumulation has been known to cause disorientation, coma, and even death. On most high-protein diets, normally healthy individuals require large amounts of water to flush this poison out of their bodies. On Stillman's Doctor's Quick Weight Loss Diet, a high-protein diet similar to Tarnower's, the dieter is required to drink at least eight 10-ounce glasses of water each day, plus as much coffee or tea and non-carbonated beverages as desired. "Drinking a lot of water," Tarnower comments, "is usually a good habit."

• Other high-protein diets with no built-in irrigation safeguards draw heavily on the body's own vital water reserves, leading to dehydration, a malady that in extreme cases can shut down the kidneys and cause death. Couple this kind of high-protein diet with jogging (or any other exercise), and the lack of water can prevent you from dissipating body heat through sweat, making you a candidate for heat stroke. Among high-school football players who beef themselves up on protein, dehydration-induced heat stroke each year produces a significant number of casualties, including deaths.

• A high-protein, low-carbohydrate diet can interfere with the normal metabolism of fats, resulting in the production of poisonous breakdown products called ketones. (Metabolism is the process by which the body utilizes foods.) To preserve bodily health, ketones, like uric acid, must be flushed out through the kidneys (more about ketones in the section on the Atkins Diet which follows). Protein metabolism is disturbed, as well, producing ammonia, a nerve toxin and cell-killer which also increases susceptibility to viral infection.

• Other investigators suggest a possible link between a high-protein diet and artery blockage, since blood cholesterol zooms upward in laboratory animals on high-protein diets even when no cholesterol is ingested.

The Tarnower Diet contains a plethora of DON'T EAT's. They include caffeine-high tea, coffee, and colas (Tarnower permits all diet sodas); non-caloric sugar substitutes which are suspected carcinogens; high-cholesterol shellfish, high-cholesterol/high-fat egg yolks, cheeses, nuts, and tuna and salmon packed in oil and salt; high-salt (sodium) pickles, olives, horseradish, instant soup mixes, canned and frozen vegetables, and club soda; pepper; and high-sugar/high-salt ketchup, soy sauce, chili sauce, and other condiments.

Although Tarnower decries the use of table salt and sugar, salt is an ingredient in many of his recipes, and sugar is an essential in his recipe for protein bread.

Tarnower bans nutritionally beneficial complex carbohydrates, including potatoes, sweet potatoes, yams, corn, peas, beans, lentils; and all baking flours other than gluten. Honey is also forbidden. The exclusion of these carbohydrate foods often tends to lower blood-sugar levels, occasionally resulting, Tarnower admits, in a draggy and dizzy feeling after a few days on the diet. Tarnower also frankly warns his readers that "Chances are you could remain on [the basic diet] without any ill effects . . . but I recommend you should not remain on [it] for more than two weeks at a time."

All in all, the Tarnower Diet does not get a clean bill of health.

Can you stay on it? Tarnower calls his diet recipes "Gourmet and International." But none of his dishes has a foreign accent, and all of his dishes are banal. The recipes are simple—so simple that results are predictably monotonous.

He uses no oil, so food can't be browned before sautéing—a simple technique that enhances the flavors of meat, chicken, pancakes, French toast, and so on. He sautés in broth, and that's fine if you like soggy, rather than crisp, food; or he sautés dry, thus toughening some foods. (For dry sautéing, he sprays his skillet before cooking with a non-stick plastic which is a suspected carcinogen.)

He is the first to bring the ersatz taste of fast foods to diet cooking. (His menus contain some deli products, as well.) The natural flavors of his foods are deadened by the overuse of salt, pepper, synthetic sweetener, and commercial sauces, including Worcestershire and tabasco. As a sop to the gourmet, he uses herbs, but the ones he uses are mostly mundane, and he uses them sparsely and uninterestingly.

Nutrition-packed, low-calorie carbohydrates—like potatoes and breads similar to mine—provide you with those feelings of fullness, lack of deprivation, and well-being which are so necessary on a low-calorie diet. But Tarnower uses no potatoes—one of the great delights of the table; you can do so many wonderful things with them. And he uses no bread except his high-protein loaf (or equivalent)—a gummy, tasteless soybean derivative. What he does use to give you a feeling of eating well is fancy names (and that's about as fancy as his recipes go).

If you're a fast-food lover, and if you can do without potatoes, bread, and other complex carbohydrates, you may be able to stay on the Tarnower Diet. But if your tastes are discerning, the chances are you'll become a Tarnower dropout.

Here's the score:

THE TARNOWER HIGH-PROTEIN DIET

	NO	MAYBE	YES
DOES IT WORK?			☑
IS IT HEALTHFUL?	☑		
CAN YOU STAY ON IT?		☑	

And on that score, it's rejected.

What's Wrong with the Atkins Diet?

"For over 50 years," reads an ad for Atkins' best-selling *Dr. Atkins' Diet Revolution,* "we've all been brainwashed into thinking that the only way to lose weight was to cut calories. 'It's a hoax!' says Dr. Robert C. Atkins. . . . [On the Atkins Diet] most men lose 7 to 8 pounds the first week . . . most women 5 to 6 pounds. . . . Have two fried eggs and all the bacon you can eat! Have chicken Kiev dripping with melted butter . . . ! You don't count calories."

On the Atkins Diet for the first two weeks, you don't have to. During that period, this extremely high-fat diet doesn't permit even a suspicion of a carbohydrate, and excess water cascades out of the body.

Does it work? For the first two weeks it works magnificently. You can actually up your caloric intake with (the ad again) "whipped cream, fried foods, cheeseburgers, all kinds of meats, poultry and seafood—even asparagus with real Hollandaise sauce!"—and still lose five pounds or more. The weight you gain in body fat is small compared to the amount you lose in body water.

But after the first two weeks, there's a sudden plunge into caloric reality. After excess water has drained off, the only way to drop weight is to drop calorie intake. Atkins permits about 1,500 calories a day. On a high-fat diet, that's not very much food. (Fats contribute about nine calories a gram; protein and carbohydrates about four each. So a high-fat diet contains less grams—less amount of food— than a high-protein, high-carbohydrate, or normal diet with the same calorie content.) The dieter goes from an overfull to a growling belly overnight.

Moreover, superfat foods to which the dieter had become accustomed during the first two weeks—the fried bacon and eggs and the whipped cream and the chicken Kiev and even the Hollandaise— are banished from the menus. They would consume so large a portion of the daily lean caloric budget that there would be little left to eat for the rest of the day. Here's a typical day's menu for the post-two-week honeymoon period as reported by a 46-year-old male Atkins disciple:

Breakfast. A cheese omelette (two eggs). A glass of seltzer.
Lunch. Two cheeseburgers (without bread). A small wedge of lettuce with oil-and-vinegar dressing. Two glasses of water.
Dinner. Broiled fish. A wedge of lettuce (no dressing). A low-calorie gelatin pudding.
Bedtime snack. Chunks of cheese.

But even though the glamour is gone, if you weigh as much as most Americans, you can continue to lose weight on Atkins' 1,500-calorie Diet. However, if you're a woman weighing under 128 or a man weighing under 125, you can't. You need less than 1,500 calories a day to keep your weight steady; so on a 1,500-calorie-a-day diet, you'll gain weight. For Harold at 125 pounds, with a weight goal of 110, the Atkins Diet was useless. And dangerous.

Is it healthful? The daily menu of Atkins' 46-year-old male disciple contained 1 percent carbohydrates, 38 percent protein, and a phenomenal 61 percent fat. (After the first two weeks, Atkins permits 1 to 3 percent carbohydrates.) The fat comes almost entirely from animal sources and is highly saturated. The preponderance of scientific evidence indicates that an extremely high-fat/high-saturated-fat diet can lead to heart attack and other degenerative diseases.

Atkins nevertheless holds that his diet is safe. He contends that the fat in his diet is burned up (oxidized) rapidly and thus rendered harmless, and that potentially harmful fat stored by the body is destroyed. The weight loss during the first two weeks, he explains, is not caused by the release of water, but by the action of a fat mobilizing hormone, F.M.H. Triggered by a zero or near-zero carbohydrate diet, it breaks down stored body fat into ketones which are eliminated from the body in the urine. But the assertion by the American Medical Association that "no such hormone has been unequivocally identified in man" may lead the objective observer to the conclusion that the Atkins Diet simply doesn't hold water.

But ketones *are* produced, and in such large amounts that they spill out of the blood into the urine, which indicates ketosis, a pathological condition found among some diabetics. Diabetes is a disease caused by the body's inability to metabolize carbohydrates. In advanced stages of the disease, only an extremely small amount of ingested carbohydrate is utilized, so the body is operating on near-zero carbohydrates, much as it does on the Atkins Diet. These advanced stages—simulated in respect to carbohydrate utilization by the Atkins Diet—are characterized by ketosis.

Ketosis can cause foul breath (the sickly smell of acetone), nausea, vomiting, apathy, menstrual aberrations, fatigue, dizziness, and weakness. It can overload the kidneys; and in persons with kidney disease, it can induce fatal kidney failure. Ketosis is also associated with increased uric acid levels, a pathway to gout.

When the body operates on near-zero carbohydrates, fat metabolism is disturbed in another way: triglycerides are produced. These are fatty substances known to be present in excess among many victims of cardiovascular diseases. (Diabetics are particularly prone to these diseases.) On the Atkins Diet, further potential danger to the heart and arteries can come from excessive quantities of salt (high blood pressure) and cholesterol (atherosclerosis). The Atkins Diet, it seemed to us, could be a cardiac time bomb.

It's a small wonder that the Committee of Public Health of the Medical Society of the County of New York denounced the Atkins Diet as "unscientific . . . unbalanced . . . and potentially dangerous."

The Atkins Diet uses all DON'T EAT's except sugar (a carbohydrate), ketchup (it contains 14.4 grams of carbohydrates per two-ounce serving), and milk (because it contains lactose, a milk sugar, which is a carbohydrate). Curiously, Atkins uses cream, which is a part of milk, and a caloric sweetener containing dextrins, simple sugars.

Because of his ban on milk, his diet may not contain enough calcium; and this, by Atkins' own admission, may lead, on occasion, to leg cramps. He treats this excruciatingly painful complaint with calcium supplements and vitamins E and C, sometimes adding doses of magnesium and potassium. A glass or so of non-fat skim milk a day would be a much simpler solution.

In magazine articles, Atkins recommended staying on his diet for only 10 to 16 days. That could have been his own answer to "Is it healthy?"

Can you stay on it? Can you imagine breads, rolls, and noodles made *without flour*? On the Atkins Diet these culinary freaks are offered with a straight face. Rolls are made with egg yolks, stiffly beaten egg whites, and an artificial sweetener; that's it. Bread is made with the same ingredients plus soy powder. And noodles are prepared with just egg and salt. They taste as horrible as they sound.

When Atkins is not being cute with his imitation baked goods, he's being heavy-handed with his other foods. His dishes are soggy with butter, cream, and cheese; spiced coarsely with salt and bacon (or, worse, with synthetic bacon bits); and overdosed with eggs. Here's how he converts a simple chicken salad into a fat-filled nightmare: chicken, celery, ¼ cup mayonnaise. . . . Isn't that fat enough? But, oh, no. He adds ¼ cup sour cream and an egg! Atkins' recipes have all the leaden qualities of the worst of East European cooking, and none of its down-to-earth goodness.

Atkins' dishes are fat-lovers' dreams-come-true. But not even the most ardent fat devotee can stomach fat as a steady diet. The English nutritionist Dr. John Yudkin allowed dieters all the fat and protein they could eat, nothing else, and found that after only a few days they couldn't force down even half of the calories they had formerly eaten. Perhaps *that's* the real secret of the Atkins Diet: the food is just too ugh-ly to swallow. No joy here.

Here's the score:

THE ATKINS HIGH-FAT DIET

	NO	MAYBE	YES
DOES IT WORK?	☐	☑	☐
IS IT HEALTHFUL?	☑	☐	☐
CAN YOU STAY ON IT?	☑	☐	☐

It scores below the Tarnower Diet, and is rejected.

What's Wrong with the Pritikin Diet?

This extremely high carbohydrate diet was invented by Mr. Nathan S. Pritikin originally for severe cardiac and angina patients, and victims of other degenerative diseases. Pritikin's basic premise is this: Since degenerative diseases are caused by fats, cholesterol, proteins, and refined carbohydrates (sugar is an example), then replacing these nutrients as far as possible with healthful complex carbohydrates (vegetables, fruits, legumes, and grains) should prevent, retard, or cure those diseases. With patients at his Longevity Center in Santa Barbara, California, his premise seems to have proved correct, as attested to by a dramatic history of successes.

Does it work as a reducing diet? On the Pritikin Diet there is no rapid weight loss in the first two weeks, as there is on the Tarnower and Atkins Diet, and, to a lesser extent, on the Diet for Life. Under clinically supervised conditions at his Longevity Center, and with the diet reinforced by a program of exercise, patients lose in a four-week stay an average of about 13 pounds—a little over three pounds a week.

It's not hard to see why. Pritikin's basic diet supplies a meager 600 calories a day, his back-up diet a scant 1,000. (An independent estimate puts the average calorie count for both diets at 666.) To understand the effects of a 600-calorie, extremely high-carbohydrate diet, consider that during the siege of Bataan in World War II, rations were cut to 1,300 to 2,000 calories a day, mainly rice (a complex carbohydrate), and the besieged were reduced to skin and bones in just a few months. On 600 calories a day, a pygmy could lose weight.

Pritikin's is not the only, nor the first, extremely low-calorie/high-carbohydrate diet. In Durham, North Carolina, famed Fat City, at any time, 315 to 470 dieters participate in Dr. Walter Kempner's rice diet, Dr. Richard Stuelke's Thin for Life Clinic's regimen, or Dr. Gerald Musante's Structure House program. And how do the dieters, who spend upward of $6.5 million a year, react? "They get a little temperamental at times," remarked a Fat City motel manager. "Anybody starving to death is going to be hard to handle."

Is it healthful? Semi-starvation diets, low in fats and cholesterol, can be. Among German prisoners of war on such diets in Russian prison camps during World War II, atherosclerosis dropped to almost nil.

But below a minimum daily caloric intake, healthful effects can be offset by harmful ones. According to findings of the U.S. Departments of Agriculture and Health, Education, and Welfare, diets of less than 800 calories a day can be dangerous to some people. Among the suspected complications are kidney stones and disturbing personality changes.

The Pritikin Diet contains 10 to 15 percent protein, 5 to 10 percent fat, and 80 percent carbohydrates, mostly complex. The low figures for fat and protein, and the whoppingly high figure for carbohydrates raise disturbing questions.

Does the Pritikin dieter get enough fat?
While the body makes its own fats (with the exception of linoleic acid fats), not enough is known about the manufacturing process to pin down accurately what raw materials the body needs and in what quantities. So there's no certainty that this lopsidedly high-carbohydrate diet can supply the necessary raw materials in the right amounts.

A too-meager amount of fats in the body could disrupt the efficient utilization of fat-soluble vitamins A, D, E, and K, with the consequences of flagging energy and general feelings of malaise. It also could deprive the body of optimum quantities of essential fatty acids, components of fats essential to the functioning of every cell in the body. Dry, scaly skin is a blatant symptom of dietary fat deprivation.

Does the Pritikin dieter get enough protein?
Pritikin's 10 to 15 percent protein allowance—call it 12.5 percent on average—is almost the same as the 12 percent recommended by the Federal Dietary Guidelines. But on a 600-calorie diet, 12.5 percent amounts to about 16 grams of protein, substantially lower than the Recommended Daily Allowance of 56 grams for men and 46 grams for women.

When insufficient protein is coupled with an extremely low-calorie diet, not only undesirable fat is reduced, but so is the vital protein in muscles and organs. Signs of subnormal protein intake include softening nails, brittle, damaged hair, dizziness, and a frustrating inability to concentrate.

Does the Pritikin dieter get too much carbohydrates?

The four-week program at Pritikin's Longevity Center is reported to reduce blood pressure, blood cholesterol, lipids (fats), triglycerides, and uric acid. That's excellent. But it often takes 20 years or more for a disease caused by a nutritional imbalance to manifest itself, and the long-range effects of this extremely high-carbohydrate diet is still to be evaluated.

So far, only one possible hazard has been determined. Since the Pritikin Diet is essentially a vegetarian diet, it could lead to pernicious anemia due to the lack of vitamin B_{12} which is only obtainable in nature through animal products. Pritikin is firmly set against the use of vitamin supplements.

Does the Pritikin dieter get enough cholesterol?

The Pritikin Diet allows less than 100 milligrams of cholesterol a day, less than either the safety-zone limitation of 160 to 185 milligrams established by one team of researchers, or the 300 milligrams recommended by the Federal Dietary Guidelines.

The body normally manufactures cholesterol to meet its needs (cholesterol is a functional component of every cell), but whether it can be produced in sufficient quantity on a 600-calorie, extremely high-carbohydrate diet has not yet been the subject of scientific investigation. The most important function of cholesterol is to supply the electrical insulation for the delicate network of the brain and the nervous system. Should the body manufacture subnormal quantities of cholesterol, and should the amount ingested be too small to bring the total amount up to normal, then the entire mechanism governing our thinking, feeling, and reflexes could be affected.

Sugar and virtually all our other DON'T EAT's (plus some of Pritikin's own) are excluded from the Pritikin Diet. But, surprisingly, a moderate amount of salt—about 2,000 to 4,000 milligrams a day—is permitted. (The body needs only about 1,100 milligrams, about 1/7 of a teaspoon.) The salt doesn't come from the shaker—that's *verboten*—but from hidden sources, like canned vegetables and overdoses of baking soda. Salt clings to water, just as carbohydrates do, and the combination of the two nutrients may cause the body to retain more than a harmless amount of excess water.

Pritikin also uses pepper, which, some nutritionists claim, can raise blood pressure; and he approves of commercial pita bread, which often is loaded with salt and undesirable fillers.

Although the Pritikin Diet is built on a solid foundation—low-fat, low-cholesterol, no sugar, and moderate amounts of salt—it goes to extremes, which could pose unsolved health problems, particularly those concerned with the effects of his restrictions over many years. Predominantly a healthful diet during its four-week application at Pritikin's Longevity Center, its long-range impact is still to be assessed.

Can you stay on it? It's not easy even to start on it, "because," Pritikin admits, "its menus are so different from what you're used to." Here's a typical daily menu:

> *Breakfast.* Cooked oatmeal plus bran. Non-fat milk. Half an orange.
> *Lunch.* Vegetable soup. Raw bell peppers, carrots, cauliflower, and cucumber.
> *Dinner.* Tomato-rice soup. Stuffed eggplant. Raw shredded cabbage, onions, and tomatoes.

And at all times the dieter is cautioned to "carry a bag filled with raw vegetables and eat them all day long. . . . If you don't . . . you run the risk of going off the diet." This is basically a vegetarian diet (meat and fish are employed as flavorings).

No wonder most people find the Pritikin Diet so different.

Pritikin recipes are flat, insipid, and so appetite-deadening that some Pritikin dieters tell us they can't swallow enough food to sustain themselves after they've reduced to ideal weight, and they continue to lose pounds. Here's my criticism of the Pritikin cuisine:

- He uses herbs uncreatively, too often relying upon dried oregano which is not particularly flavorsome. He makes little use of garlic—that wonder herb—and when he does include it in a recipe, it's only in sparing amounts. He prefers garlic powder, a pallid substitute. His dominant seasoning is pepper, but miraculously his dishes remain bland in spite of it. On the whole, he uses his seasonings in insufficient amounts to titillate the taste buds.
- He sautées in broth or water, producing soggy, rather than crisp, dishes. Always cooked without oil, his vegetables, and the minute amount of meat and fish he permits, lack texture, flavor, and character. His solid cooked food comes to the table as if it had been drenched with a garden hose.
- His saltless soups, made with water, not stock, and with only a smattering of mismatched herbs, are worse than their hospital counterparts.
- His salad dressings—combinations of vinegar, water, and herbs—are soups rather than dressings—which is fine if you like your salads awash in vinegar broth.
- He makes heavy use of beaten egg whites, which convert already bland dishes into even blander ones.

- His bread, which is made from water, whole wheat flour, and too much yeast, is coarse, dry, and tasteless.
- He includes few cakes, and very few desserts, none of which is exciting.
- He appears to let his own taste preferences sometimes override his sense of nutritional prudence. Nova Scotia lox fin is a prized delicacy, but it's egregiously high in fat. And why lox in the first place? It's smoked salmon, and smoked products are salty and may contain suspected carcinogens.
- Going through Pritikin's recipes, I sense overall an unwholesome underlying theme: you have to suffer to be healthy.

Add all this suffering at the table—and away from it with that filled-up plastic bag of raw vegetables—to a near-starvation allowance of 600 calories a day, and it seems unlikely that anybody outside the walls of the Longevity Center could stay on the Pritikin Diet without possessing monumental motivation.

Here's the score:

THE PRITIKIN HIGH-CARBOHYDRATE DIET

	NO	MAYBE	YES
DOES IT WORK?	☐	☐	☑

But slowly

IS IT HEALTHFUL?	☐	☑	☐
CAN YOU STAY ON IT?	☐	☑	☐

If you're very motivated

It has many advantages, it's far superior to the Tarnower and Atkins Diets, but it's not for us.

CAUTION: so far as my critique of the Pritikin Diet, or any other diet, is concerned—*remember that it's based on my opinion and my husband's.* Armed with facts, including your doctor's advice, and with your own dietary experience, you should come to your own conclusions. Any diet that works for you, and on which you're healthy and happy, is a good diet *for you.*

What's Wrong with the Prudent Diet?

Dr. Norman Jolliffe was director of the New York City Department of Nutrition when, convinced that the rich American diet was directly responsible for the national epidemic of heart attack and other degenerative diseases, he developed his corrective and preventive Prudent Diet. In 1958, he decided to put his new diet to the test.

Through newspaper ads, he recruited volunteers—Jolliffe's famous 400 human guinea pigs—and enrolled them into his Anti-Coronary Club. To retain their membership, they had to live on a diet low in cholesterol and fats, particularly saturated fats, and devoid of—Jolliffe invented this term—"empty calories." Empty calories are contributed by denatured foods—foods which have been robbed by commercial processing of their vitamins, minerals, and other natural nutrients. Among empty calorie foods are sugar (sucrose), highly refined and unenriched white flour, saturated fats, and almost all commercially prepared foods, particularly baked products.

In 1962, four years after the experiment began, Jolliffe announced the results to the New York Medical Society. On a normal American diet, 25 of the 400 human guinea pigs might have been expected to have had heart attacks. On the Prudent Diet, only four heart attacks occurred. The Prudent Diet decreased the incidence of heart attack by an amazing 650 percent!

In subsequent years, Anti-Coronary Clubs spread throughout the nation. The success of the original club was not only replicated, but evidence piled up to demonstrate that the Prudent Diet helped forestall or reverse a catalog of other degenerative diseases, including atherosclerosis, diabetes, gout, cataracts, yellow atrophy of the liver, and exotic lipid diseases, the symptoms of which are fat-and-cholesterol bumps on various parts of the body. Not too low or too high in basic nutrient percentages—about 20 percent fat, 25 percent protein, and 55 percent carbohydrates—this diet prudently avoided the hazards of extreme nutrient imbalance associated with other diets.

As a reducing diet, it worked well. The average daily menu contributed a satisfying 1,500 calories. His cuisine, packed with tasty forbidden foods, rated at least one star. It featured such dishes as green salad with lemon-sherry sauce, New England clam chowder, turkey with oyster stuffing and cranberry relish, vegetables in aspic, and *blanc mange* and flan. Little or no sense of deprivation here.

But the Prudent Diet had four major drawbacks. The basic nutrient breakdown didn't reflect recent advances in nutritional biochemistry. As salutory as the diet was, it contained too many potentially unhealthful ingredients, chief among which was salt. Without those ingredients (many of our DON'T EAT's), the cuisine was inedible. And the diet provided no fast initial weight loss—a must to encourage the dieter.

So the score was less than perfect:

THE JOLLIFFE PRUDENT DIET

	NO	MAYBE	YES
DOES IT WORK?	☐	☐	☑
			But slowly
IS IT HEALTHFUL?	☐	☑	☐
CAN YOU STAY ON IT?	☐	☐	☑
			But not with
			DON'T EAT's removed

We decided to make it meet all three criteria.

Our first task was to bring the basic nutrient breakdown up to date. We did that by making small adjustments in the protein and carbohydrate percentages. Here is—

How the Diet for Life Compares with Other Diets and Government Guidelines *

COMPARISON OF THE MAJOR DIET PLANS

	Fat	Protein	Carbohydrates
Doctor's (1950) high-protein/high-fat	59.5	33	7.5
Tarnower high-protein	22.5	43	34.5
Atkins high-fat	61–62	31	0–1
Pritikin high-carbohydrate	5–10	10–15	80
Jolliffe (1959) balanced	20	25	55
Diet for Life balanced	20	20	60
Federal Dietary Guidelines balanced	30	12	58

* The *Diet for Life* complies more closely to Federal Dietary Guidelines than any other diet charted. It is also the lowest in salt content, and the second lowest on cholesterol content, averaging about 160 milligrams a day. Charted nutrients are expressed in percentages of total daily caloric intake.

We overcame, one by one, the three other drawbacks of the Prudent Diet. You already know from the previous chapter how we eliminated the DON'T EAT's, and how I created an haute cuisine of health using only healthful ingredients. You'll find out how we overcame the final drawback—the lack of fast initial weight loss—in the chapter that follows.

The score for our modified version of the Prudent Diet became:

THE DIET FOR LIFE

	NO	MAYBE	YES
DOES IT WORK?	☐	☐	☑
IS IT HEALTHFUL?	☐	☐	☑
CAN YOU STAY ON IT?	☐	☐	☑

4

Drop Eight Pounds or More in the First Two Weeks— without Sacrificing a Calorie

Your Ideal Weight

CHART OF IDEAL WEIGHTS *

Height	MEN Build				WOMEN Build		
(feet and inches)	light	medium	heavy		light	medium	heavy
4–10	95	100	105		90	94	98
4–11	97	103	108		93	98	102
5–0	100	106	111		95	100	105
5–1	105	111	117		97	102	108
5–2	110	117	123		100	106	111
5–3	115	122	128		105	112	118
5–4	120	127	133		110	116	123
5–5	125	132	138		112	119	126
5–6	130	137	143		117	124	130
5–7	133	141	148		120	127	134
5–8	137	145	153		125	132	139
5–9	143	151	159		130	137	144
5–10	148	156	164		135	142	149
5–11	152	160	168		140	147	154
6–0	155	163	171		144	151	158
6–1	163	171	179				
6–2	167	175	183				
6–3	170	179	188				
6–4	172	181	195				
6–5	178	188	198				
6–6	185	195	206				

* Compiled from statistics prepared by the U.S. Department of Agriculture; H.E.W. Conference, 1973; and various medical and insurance company studies

If you're 10 percent over your ideal weight—obese by definition—each additional pound can cost you a month of your life, according to insurance company statistics. If your ideal weight is 120 and you weigh 146, you could be shortening your life expectancy by a year. It's senseless when you can reduce in just two easy steps.

In *Step 1,* you can drop excess water weight fast, about eight pounds in two weeks, without impaired fat metabolism and induced ketosis.

In *Step 2,* you can cut excess fat weight as fast as three pounds a week without any sense of deprivation caused by near-starvation or unappetizing diets.

You can get started on *Step 1* without the sudden low-calorie shock of other diets. And you can continue to lose water weight while eating as many calories—but more healthful calories—as you had been eating right along. The secret is simple:

Just cut out *all* added salt: the salt on your table, in your cooking, and hidden in almost every kind of commercial food you buy in supermarkets, delicatessens, take-out places, and restaurants. On the superbly seasoned Diet for Life, you'll never miss the salt.

We discovered this fast, safe method of water-weight loss serendipitously.

Fighting High Blood Pressure

We were looking for a way to cut down high blood pressure (hypertension), the silent killer associated with many degenerative diseases, the deadliest of which is heart attack. When diastolic pressure (the low figure on the blood-pressure report) goes from 60 to 70, the risk of heart attack doubles; it doubles again from 70 to 85; and it doubles once more from 85 to 100. When the diastolic pressure reaches 110, the chance of heart attack has escalated by a terrifying 800 percent.

Among the 15 to 20 percent of the nation who are genetically prone to high blood pressure, the disease can be brought on by a high-salt diet. Since it's impossible to know in advance of hypertensive symptoms whether you are among that 15-to-20-percent, it's wise to take no risks and switch to a low-salt diet. The diet could also help prevent high-salt-induced impairment of fat metabolism, another pathway to degenerative diseases.

Certainly, we thought, Harold's cardiologist would insist he go on a low-salt diet. But he didn't. (In the hospital, Harold's food was amply salted, and unlimited quantities of salt were available at every meal.) Instead, he prescribed Hydrodiuril, a diuretic which forces the kidneys to flush out water, thus carrying away excess salt. (Actually, what's carried away is sodium. Salt, sodium chloride, is a combination of the chemicals sodium and chlorine. Of the two, sodium is the more important biochemically. It's the excess of sodium which leads to pathological conditions.)

The diuretic also flushes out essential vitamins and minerals, particularly potassium, a deficiency of which affects the ability of the muscles, including the heart muscle, to contract. Drugs of the Hydrodiuril type have also been known to hasten the onset of diabetes, and increase the blood levels of gout-inducing uric acid. Used consistently, these drugs can flush out too much sodium, resulting in "the low-salt syndrome" characterized by nausea, dizziness, weakness often to the point of collapse, and sometimes coma, which may lead to death.

The worst indictment against the use of a diuretic to treat high blood pressure is this—*it does not cure.* Once the use of the drug is stopped, blood pressure returns to its former high level. (In some cases the level is higher than before the use of the drug.) To control high blood pressure by means of Hydrodiuril can mean a commitment to the drug for the rest of your life. To Harold and to me, this was a repugnant prospect.

It seemed to us there was a simple, safe alternative way to normalize high blood pressure due to excess salt: simply cut down on salt intake.

Some medical evidence supported our conclusion. In the '60s an American research team found that a low-salt diet was as effective in controlling hypertension as Hydrodiuril-type drugs. The finding was corroborated in the '70s by Australian medical researchers. In addition, the scientists discovered that a low-salt diet, provided the daily salt intake was kept above a basic minimum, could not produce the low-salt syndrome or any other diuretic-induced side effect.

When we decided to switch over to a low-salt diet, we learned about its weight-reducing effects. Excess salt in the body soaks up water like a sponge. As long as the body is fed excess salt, it holds excess water. Most of us carry around as much as eight pounds of salt-related water with us, and some of us as much as 16. When salt intake is reduced, you reduce.

How Much Salt Is Right for You?

Salt is measured in milligrams of sodium. (There are 454 grams in a pound, and a milligram is $\frac{1}{1,000}$ of a gram.) A teaspoon of salt weighs about 7,000 milligrams (7 grams), and it contains about 2,800 milligrams of sodium (2.8 grams).

The normal amount of sodium needed by the body is only about 220 to 400 milligrams a day. Doctors who treat hypertension without drugs recommend a sodium intake of less than 500 milligrams a day.

Recommendations from government sources are higher: about 1,200 to 2,000 milligrams a day.

Our basic nutritional strategy is conservatism. Since the body needs at the most 400 milligrams of sodium a day, and hypertension is treated with under 500 milligrams a day, we play it safe and set 500 milligrams as our maximum daily intake. On the Diet for Life, you'll get no more sodium than that—and you'll get it from wholesome, unprocessed foods which naturally contain small amounts of sodium.

How Much Weight Does Excess Sodium Put on You?

On 400 milligrams of sodium a day, your body is likely to be free of unnecessary salt-retained water. As a rule of thumb, you hold on to two pounds of excess water for 1,000 milligrams consumed over 400. If you're an average American, you consume about 4,300 milligrams of sodium a day (equivalent to about 10,000 milligrams of salt, about 1½ teaspoons), and consequently cling to about eight pounds of water you don't need.

Where does excess water come from? Salt increases thirst, and you drink a great deal (bartenders don't serve salted peanuts just to please your palate). There's also a lot of of water in every bite of food you eat; and salt holds onto it. Chinese food—often recommended by diet doctors because it's low in fat, cholesterol, and calories—is so high in sodium (particularly when M.S.G., monosodium glutamate, is added) that you can get up from a simple meal in a Chinese restaurant two to three pounds heavier than when you sat down. It's happened to us. (Watch out for Japanese food. It's the saltiest in the world.)

Excess salt can also put fat on you. By increasing the flow of saliva, it stimulates a desire—virtually a compulsion—to eat more. That's why you've never tasted an appetizer that wasn't salty (except one of mine). And that's why you can't stop eating potato chips, or any other commercially prepared snack. One researcher reported to a meeting of the American Medical Association that potato chip and pretzel addicts can often gain as much as three pounds of fat a day.

We're a nation of overweight people not only because we eat too much, but because we eat too much salt.

Less Salt Can Cut Pre-Menstrual Weight Gain, and Ease Other Monthly Miseries

Many women gain as much as five pounds during their pre-menstrual periods. The weight gain is often associated with feeling bloated, headachy, draggy, crochety, and weepy. Some women even fly into irrational rages; and many husbands and wives have had their most bitter disputes during this time. The villain behind pre-menstrual weight gain and accompanying miseries has recently been identified by medical research teams as excess salt.

To wash out the excess salt, one leading woman diet doctor prescribes diuretics. Although many women don't know it, most non-prescription pre-menstrual medications are mainly diuretics combined with aspirin and caffeine. But diuretics not only wash out salt; they drain the body of potassium, magnesium, and B vitamins, as well, which could intensify your pre-menstrual miseries. The B vitamins are needed to help fight irritability and emotional distur-bances, and potassium and magnesium are required to help combat that draggy feeling.

The drug-free, and often more effective way, to control the effects of excess salt during the pre-menstrual period is to sharply curtail your intake of salt. On the Diet for Life, I've experienced no weight gain and none of the other monthly symptoms many women antici-pate with dread. (Woman-to-woman hint: don't wear pantyhose or tight girdles during your pre-menstrual period. They trap water, and therefore prevent its elimination.)

Less Salt Can Make You More Attractive

Excess salt puts on weight in the wrong places. We tried an experi-ment on ourselves to prove our low-salt diet could get the weight off those places—and fast.

We decided to eat dinner for five consecutive nights in two- and three-star restaurants. We told the waiter to remove the salt shaker from the table, and we ordered only those dishes which most Amer-icans regard as non-salty. Most important: we ate no more calories than we would have eaten on the Diet for Life.

Yet at the end of five days, each of us had gained four pounds. The weight gain had resulted from the hidden salt in the "non-salty" dishes. (And this was in top-flight restaurants. Beginning on page 68, I'll tell you about the even more staggering amounts of hidden salt contained in the dishes prepared at ordinary restaurants.)

A good deal of the excess weight went to our faces. My skin puffed up and looked unhealthy, and so did Harold's. The areas under our eyes were bloated. We looked as if we had just tumbled out of bed after a sleepless night. We seemed to have aged.

When we returned to three meals a day on the Diet for Life, the excess water drained away in four days. Back to ideal weight. No more puffiness. Firm and healthy-looking skin. No swelling under our eyes. We were rejuvenated.

The experiment was a success.

Try a similar experiment when you switch from your current high-salt diet to the Diet for Life. Take a snapshot of yourself before you start. Scotch-tape it to your bathroom mirror. Then, after two weeks on the diet, look in the mirror and compare yourself with the snapshot. Chances are, *you* will be more attractive.

A Guide to Hidden Salt in Supermarket Foods

Our experience with "non-salty" food in two- and three-star restaurants emphasizes the dangers of hidden salt. There's salt hidden in every food that's canned, jarred, bottled, boxed, frozen, pre-baked, or processed in any way. (The exceptions are products labeled "No salt added.") There's even salt in sweets. Salt is the nation's No. 2 processed-food additive. (Sugar is No. 1.)

Here is a list of supermarket foods which contain hidden salt. (It's arranged alphabetically.) Read the list carefully before you go shopping. There are some shocking surprises in store for you.

SUPERMARKET FOODS CONTAINING HIDDEN SALT

Anchovies

Baked goods
 An English muffin contains 293 milligrams of sodium; a slice of enriched white bread, 161; of whole-wheat bread, 211; of pie, 414.
Baking mixes, including quick-rising
Baking powder
Baking soda
Barbecue sauce
Bouillon cubes
Butter, salted
Breakfast foods
 Most standard-brand breakfast foods contain 260 to 370 milligrams of sodium per serving.
Buttermilk, salted.

Cakes and cookies
 An average-sized cookie contains 178 milligrams of sodium; Twinkies has 210.
Candy
 Salt makes sugar taste sweeter. An average-sized candy bar contains about 68 milligrams of sodium.
Canned foods
 They're very heavily salted. Asparagus are naturally low in sodium, 3.5 milligrams per serving, but canned asparagus contain 560 milligrams per serving.
Caviar
Celery flakes
Celery salt
Cereals, quick-cooking
Cereals, breakfast
 See Breakfast foods.
Cheeses

Chili sauce
Chinese food, frozen
   Even if M.S.G. is omitted, the food will be high in salt because most Chinese
   dishes are made with highly salted chicken stock.
Chocolate, instant mixes
Chocolate milk
Cocoa, instant mixes
Cookies
   See Cakes and cookies.
Corned meats
   "Corned" means salted. In England corned beef is called salt beef.
Crackers

Delicatessen
   Salt content here is even higher than canned foods. Enough ham to fill a sandwich contains 1,500 milligrams of sodium; a serving of breakfast sausages, 1,000.

Finnan haddie
Flour, self-rising
Frozen dinners and prepared dishes
   A frozen-food chicken dinner contains 1,152 milligrams of sodium.
Frozen fish fillets
Frozen lima beans
   A serving of natural lima beans contains a negligible .2 milligrams of sodium; a
   serving of frozen lima beans, has about 235.

Garlic salt
Gelatin, flavored

Horseradish, bottled

Ice cream
   About 70 milligrams per serving

Japanese foods

Ketchup
Koshered meats
   The sodium content of a serving of regular, non-kosher lean beef is about 92
   milligrams; koshered, the serving contains 2,270 milligrams. (For observant Jews
   on a restricted-salt diet, rabbinical law waives the koshering requirement.)

Lox

Margarine
Mayonnaise
Meat extracts
Meat glazes
Meats, salted
Meat sauces
Meat tenderizers
Milk, condensed or evaporated
   About 128 milligrams per eight ounces
Milk, non-fat

About 126 milligrams per eight ounces
Milk, whole
    About 122 milligrams per eight ounces
Milk drinks
Mineral waters (except low-sodium)
M.S.G. (monosodium glutamate)
Mustard

Nova Scotia salmon
Nut butters
    Peanut butter contains 178 milligrams per serving.
Nuts, salted

Olives
Onion salt
Oriental foods, processed

Pickles and pickled products
Pies
Popcorn, salted
Potato chips
Pretzels
    A quarter-pound contains 1,925 milligrams of sodium.
Pudding mixes
    A serving contains as much as 828 milligrams of sodium.

Relishes
Rennet tablets
Rolls
    See Baked goods.

Salad dressings
Sauerkraut
Seasonings with salt added
Sherbets
Smoked foods
    Smoking is a form of salting.
Soft drinks
Soups, canned
    A simple tomato soup can contain as much as 1,192 milligrams of sodium.
Soups, instant mixes
Soy sauce

Take-out foods
TV dinners
    See Frozen dinners and prepared dishes.

Worcestershire sauce
Wursts
    See Delicatessen.

Read labels, and avoid all foods containing sodium additives like sodium alginate, sodium benzoate, sodium hydroxide, sodium nitrate, sodium nitrite, sodium propionate, and sodium sulfite; the latter is often added to dry fruit as a preservative.

Hidden-salt foods are not found only in supermarkets. You can come across them anyplace processed foods are sold. When you shop in health-food stores, read the labels, especially on cakes, candies, and cereals. Watch out, too, for salt disguised as sea salt, or seaweed preparations. Sea salt is table salt plus a garnish of trace elements. Seaweed preparations, like dulse and kelp, are admittedly rich in vital minerals, particularly iodine, but are extremely high in sodium. And avoid salt substitutes; the taste is wrong.

Watch Out for Sodium in Non-Prescription Medicinals and Tap Water

Carry a copy of this list along with you the next time you visit the drugstore.

HIDDEN SODIUM IN DRUGSTORE PRODUCTS

Product	Milligrams of sodium	
Alka-Seltzer	521	per tablet
Aspirin	97	per tablet *
Bisodol powder	471	per teaspoon
Brioschi	710	per dose
Bromo-Seltzer	717	per teaspoon
Citrocarbonates	4,550	per teaspoon
Fleet's enema	300	per dose
Metamucil Instant Mix	250	per dose
Miles Nervine	544	per dose
Rolaids	53	per tablet
Sal Hepatica	1,000	per dose
Sodium bicarbonate	177	per tablet *

All antacids, analgesics, laxatives, and some cough preparations contain sodium.

---

* 300-milligram tablet

Take salt pills only on your doctor's advice. If you think salt pills are a harmless way to restore salt loss after a strenuous workout on the tennis court (or after any other kind of strenuous activity), you could be wrong, according to recent research studies. Salt-pill abuse can lead to a thickening of the blood and to loss of potassium. Thickening of the blood decreases the amount of oxygen the heart receives, making it work harder, while loss of potassium weakens the ability of the heart to contract efficiently. The results of salt-pill abuse, the studies report, can range from the harmful to the fatal.

The best way to avoid sodium in drugs is to avoid drugs altogether. (But check with your doctor first.)

All drinking water contains some sodium, usually in small amounts. But in El Paso, Texas, the sodium content of an eight-ounce glass of tap water is about 428 milligrams; in Crandall, Texas, about 400 milligrams; and throughout the Southwest, about 40 to 70 milligrams. Your local Water District Office will tell you how much sodium comes out of your tap. (For the sodium content of the drinking water in 100 large American cities, write for *Sodium in Food, Medicine and Water,* issued by the Water Quality Associates, 447 East Butterfield Road, Lombard, Illinois 60148. It's free.)

How to Cut Your Salt Intake at Home and in Restaurants

At home. Ban your salt shaker. If you're like most Americans, you shake on ½ teaspoon to 1¼ teaspoons of salt a day, which hold on to about two to five pounds of water in your body.

Ban all processed foods containing added salt. The approved list of Diet for Life foods (Chapter 2) will provide all the sodium you need.

Ban your recipes which call for salt. They add about 1,750 to 3,500 milligrams per serving to your dishes, and up to 220 milligrams to a slice of your homemade bread. (But don't throw those recipes away. In Chapter 8, I'll show you how to convert them to Diet for Life recipes.)

If instead of taking these sensible steps, you continue to consume salt as usual at home, you'll continue to lug from three to seven pounds of excess water weight around with you.

In restaurants. Except for ignoring the salt shaker, there's nothing you can do about reducing your salt consumption in fast-food restaurants. A simple lunch consisting of a cheeseburger, relish, pickle, and a cola drink fills you up with about 3,500 milligrams of sodium, which will retain about six pounds of excess water weight.

Try a diet lunch in a coffee shop, and you'll hold on to more water weight than you lose in fat weight. A salad with house dressing, a cup of tomato soup, and two graham crackers contribute about 1,900 milligrams of sodium, which is equivalent to about three pounds of excess water weight. (About canned soup as a diet food: the reliable *Consumer Reports* warns that "canned soup may be All-American, but it's not a nutritious meal." We agree. By and large, canned soups are low in proteins and polyunsaturates, and derive their carbohydrates mainly from sugar. What you're eating is essentially a high-salt broth flavored with suggestions of vegetables, meat, fish, seafood, and chicken.)

In moderate-priced-to-expensive restaurants, you can control your salt intake in the following ways:

1. Begin your meal with fresh fruit. Most restaurants offer a fresh fruit cup, no sugar added, which can be delicious. The natural sugars in the fruit will help you take the edge off your appetite, and that's a plus when you're watching calories.

2. Order a plain green salad with oil and vinegar on the side. Do not ask for oil-and-vinegar dressing, which is pre-prepared and contains salt. Hint: carry your favorite herbs or non-salt mix with you and stir it into the oil and vinegar.

3. Ask the waiter for a simple grilled steak or chop, or a broiled *whole* fish. Emphasize: *no* salt, please. For the fish, instruct the waiter: do *not* add bouillon before broiling. Here's the reason for a whole fish, rather than a fillet or steak: when you also request no butter in the cooking (as you will when you're on the Diet for Life) a fish fillet or steak will arrive on your plate dry, tough-textured, and tasteless. A whole fish, on the other hand, will retain its juices, and arrive moist, tender, and sweet-tasting. Hint: if you can't persuade the waiter to have the chef season your selection with herbs, sprinkle on herbs or a non-salt herb mix which you've brought with you.

4. For dessert, only fruit is safe. If you've already had it for a first course, skip dessert.

5. Drink fresh fruit or vegetable juices. When they're not available, settle for the canned or bottled variety, no salt or sugar added. (Avoid low-sodium Perrier-with-lime during meals. You'll find out why on page 78.)

Caution: health-food restaurants are no more sparing in their use of salt than any other kind of restaurant. If you must eat in them (and there are some reasons why not to on page 240), follow the preceding salt-control program.

Lunch is the biggest eat-out problem, and the best way to solve it is with a brown paper bag. It's become chic, it's a money-saver, and it gives you more free time (aren't you tired of sitting in a restaurant most of your lunchtime just waiting for the food and the check to arrive?). You'll find suggestions on page 90 for stuffing your brown paper bag with delectable Diet for Life delights.

Our Approved List of Commercial Low-Sodium Foods

Because of the nation's rising level of nutritional awareness, several food-processing companies in recent years have packaged a variety of products with no salt added. Regrettably, a large number of those products contain either sugar, or fat/saturated fat, or cholesterol, or combinations of these restricted ingredients; and almost all of those products fail our taste test. But there are some gems among the dross, and here they are arranged alphabetically:

HEALTHFUL COMMERCIAL LOW-SODIUM FOODS

Baking powder

Breakfast foods: shredded wheat; puffed rice, wheat, and millet; some granolas (made without sugar, coconut, or coconut and palm oils); and non-instant oatmeal and cream of wheat

Chili con carne seasoning (not the powder)
Curry powder (Be sure there's no salt added.)

Pineapple, canned, in its own juices

Salmon, canned, packed in water (not broth)

Tomato juice, canned
   It's a revelation. It tastes like freshly squeezed tomatoes.
Tomato paste
Tomato purée
Tuna, canned, packed in water (not broth)

Start Your Diet on a Food-Flavor Binge

The Diet for Life no-salt-added menus have been hailed by one syndicated columnist as "rivaling a gourmet tour of New York's upper East Side." Instead of responding to just one dominant taste—the taste of salt—your palate will experience a dazzling rainbow of flavors. Reducing with the Diet for Life is an adventure in eating.

Your object in *Step 1* of this reducing diet is to get rid of your excess water weight. You'll find a menu-and-recipe program beginning on page 81 which will do it for you.

The daily menus average about 1,250 calories, low enough to cut fat weight on most Americans. But it's far more comfortable—and puts less strain on the body—to lose water weight first, then fat weight. So—*reduce without sacrificing a calorie in the following way:*

1. Determine the amount of calories you need to maintain your present body weight by multiplying your weight by 15.
2. Add to the 1,250 calories a day on the Diet for Life reducing menus enough calories to maintain your present weight, using one or more of the following methods:
   a. Add more snacks.
   b. Add more dishes to your meals.
   c. Increase the size of servings.
   d. Substitute higher-calorie dishes for those on the menu.

IMPORTANT: use only Diet for Life recipes and Diet for Life favored ingredients (Chapter 9). You can use some of the favored ingredients for as-is snacks, and all of the favored ingredients for creating Diet for Life recipes of your own (Chapter 8). To make your calorie counting easy, caloric information is provided for all recipes and favored ingredients.

Your scale will probably begin to show weight loss on the third or fourth day of the diet. You'll continue to lose weight until all excess water has drained out of your body. You'll know that's happened when your scale shows no weight loss for two consecutive days. Harold reached steady weight in two weeks, after registering a water-weight loss of eight pounds. If you're carrying around more than eight pounds of excess water, it may take you more than two weeks to lose it; if you're carrying around less than eight pounds, it may take you less than two weeks.

Since there's an ample supply of carbohydrates in the Diet for Life, there's no chance of the impaired fat metabolism and consequent ketosis associated with low-carbohydrate, water-weight-loss diets. Following our rule of nutritional conservatism, many favored Diet for Life ingredients are high in potassium to compensate for any possible loss of that mineral as excess water is released through the kidneys. Among these high-potassium ingredients are: apples, apple juice, artichokes, asparagus, bananas, lima beans, blackberries, broccoli, Brussels sprouts, buckwheat, cabbage, carrots, cauliflower, celery, chard, cherries, chestnuts, corn, dates, lentils, mushrooms, oatmeal, onions, parsley, potatoes, raisins, dark rye flour, and whole sesame seeds.

The first two weeks or so on the Diet for Life will do more than start you on the road to a slimmer you. It will introduce you to a whole new joyous way of healthful eating. The mouth-watering cuisine is not only salt-free, but also sugar-free and low in fat/saturated fat and cholesterol. It's the same cuisine you'll enjoy for the rest of your life—for the sake of your life.

Now go on to *Step 2,* and learn how to rid yourself of your excess fat while expanding the joys of the table.

5

Lose from One to Three Pounds of Fat a Week without Feeling Deprived—and Keep It Off

You may not look fat after excess-water loss (Harold didn't), but if you're over ideal weight, you *are* fat. Conduct this test to prove it: pinch the skin over your stomach; if you're holding ½ inch or more of flesh between your fingers, almost all of it is fat.

Set your fat-weight-loss goal by subtracting your ideal weight (page 59) from your weight after excess-water loss. If you weigh 180 after excess-water loss, and your ideal weight is 165, your fat-weight-loss goal is 15 pounds (180 minus 165).

Losing those fat pounds is going to be one of the most momentous experiences of your life. Why not make a record of it? Take a large sheet of paper, and near the top of it write your fat-weight-loss goal in big red letters. Paste the paper on your full-length dressing mirror. Then when you lose your first pound of fat, draw a slash through the numeral, and write the poundage still to go under it. So 15 becomes:

$$\frac{\cancel{15}}{14}$$

As you lose each pound, continue the slash down, until 1 becomes:

$$\frac{\cancel{1}}{0}$$

And you've done it!

Watching those numbers dwindle, and at the same time seeing yourself growing slimmer in your mirror, can give you moments of exhilaration you've never felt before. At the final zero, you'll view your new trim shape with a glowing sense of achievement.

But for those rewards, you've got to give up something—calories. That's—

The Only Nutritional Way to Get Rid of Fat

Your body uses up energy: not much when you're sleeping; more when you're making love; and a lot more when you're on the tennis court. Calories are units of energy. You get your energy (calories) from food.

When your body uses up less energy (calories) than you get in your food, the excess energy is stored as fats, and you gain weight.

When your body uses up more energy (calories) than you get in your food, the stored fats are converted back into energy to make up the difference. Energy is produced when the fats are burned (as you would burn fuel in a furnace). The end products of normal fat combustion are carbon dioxide and water, which are excreted through the lungs and kidneys, respectively. The fat no longer exists, and you lose weight. There is no other nutritional way—no combinations of foodstuffs, no pills, no gastronomic magic or taboos—that will reduce your fat.

Exercise? It increases the number of calories your body needs; so if you don't increase the number of calories in your meals during the time you exercise, you will lose weight. But that's the hard way to do it. To drop a pound of fat a week without cutting food calories, you would have to run half the length of Manhattan at a brisk five and a half miles an hour for six consecutive days. It's much easier, and far more pleasant, to shrink your fat by sitting down to Diet for Life gourmet repasts. (On the other hand, don't just sit there. We're gung-ho for exercise of the right kind, and in Chapter 13, I'll tell you how we flex our muscles, and why.)

If you balk at cutting calories even on delectable food, consider what trimming away your fat will do for you. Over the long range it can block pathways to degenerative diseases by lowering blood pressure and blood lipid levels, stave off heart attack, and add years to your life and life to your years. Over the short range, it can make you feel healthier, more energetic, more alert—and, above all, it can make you feel good about yourself. Look in the mirror on zero day, and meet the new slim, bright, younger-looking, attractive you. Worth a few calories, isn't it?

How Fast Should You Lose Fat?

Would you like to be mean, surly, depressed and withdrawn? Would you like to face the possibilities of nutrient deficiencies, menstrual irregularities, infertility, hair loss, skin changes, cold intolerance, severe constipation, and other complications? If your answer is no, don't lose more than three pounds of fat a week.

How to Calculate How Fast You'll Lose Fat

The Diet for Life fat-reducing menus consist of about 1,250 calories a day. For most people that results in a fat-weight loss of from one to three pounds a week.

But you are not most people. *To calculate how much weight* you *will lose weekly* on 1,250 calories a day, apply Formula I:

1. Multiply your present weight by 15
2. Subtract 1,250
3. Multiply the result by 7
4. Divide by 3,500

If you weigh 180, this is how the formula works out:

1. $180 \times 15 = 2,700$
2. Subtract $1,250 = 1,450$
3. $1,450 \times 7 = 10,150$
4. Divide by $3,500 = 3$ pounds

Heavyweights: Reduce Fat on High Caloric Allowances

If you're on the heavy side, you could lose more than three pounds a week on 1,250 calories a day. Say you're 220. Then:

1. $220 \times 15 = 3,300$
2. Subtract $1,250 = 2,050$
3. $2,050 \times 7 = 14,350$
4. Divide by $3,500 = $ about 4 pounds

And that's one pound too many.

You have to adjust your daily caloric allowance upward to bring your fat-weight loss down to three pounds or less. How far upward? *To calculate how many calories a day* you *need to lose one, two, or three fat-pounds per week,* use Formula II:

1. Multiply your present weight by 15.
2. Multiply your desired weekly fat-weight loss—1, 2, or 3 pounds—by 500.
3. Subtract.

At 220 pounds:

1. 220 × 15 = 3,300
2. 3 × 500 = 1,500
3. Subtract = 1,800

You can consume 1,800 calories a day (not 1,250) and lose three pounds a week.

Should you desire to lose only one pound a week:

1. 220 × 15 = 3,300
2. 1 × 500 =   500
3. Subtract = 2,800

you can add another 1,000 calories a day to your allowance.

If you're heavy, you know you need a large number of calories to get through the day, and on a fixed low-calorie diet of 600 to 1,500 calories a day, you're likely to suffer more than most people. However, the Diet for Life is based not on suffering, but on joy. The heavier you are, the more calories you can consume while losing fat-weight.

How to Take Off Fat the Diet for Life Way

It's simple.

1. Determine how many pounds you'll lose on 1,250 calories a day by applying Formula I on page 74. If the formula shows you'll lose three pounds a week or less, just follow the menus in the next chapter.

2. If the formula shows you'll lose more than three pounds a week, decide on how many pounds you want to lose each week: one, two, or three. Advice: the slower you lose weight, the easier it is.

3. Determine the daily caloric allowance for your desired weight loss by applying Formula II on page 74.

4. Using the 1,250-calories-a-day daily menus as a base, add sufficient calories according to instructions on page 70 to supply your daily caloric allowance.

Lose Fat without a Sense of Deprivation

A recent Cornell University Conference on Therapy, reviewing 15 years of clinical experience in dieting, concluded: "Most persons will not stay on diets." The reasons: calorie deprivation and taste deprivation.

On the Diet for Life fat-reducing program, the dieter feels no sense of calorie-deprivation because:

There's an adequate basic daily caloric allowance of 1,250 calories. For heavier dieters, the number of calories are augmented:

1. The serving portions are ample to copious.
2. There is a sufficient amount of fiber in the diet to provide a feeling of fullness.
3. The diet is rich in complex carbohydrates which feed into the bloodstream slowly and steadily, fighting off hunger signals.
4. The menus include such satisfying foods as bread and rolls, cakes, pasta, and stunning desserts.

But calorie-deprivation is the lesser of the two diet deterrents. So well established is the repulsiveness of traditional diet food that: "As a result," one eminent nutritionist warns, "you may feel miserable during the first seven or eight days on a diet." With admirable restraint, he adds, "A bit of extra patience is valuable."

On the Diet for Life, there is no miserable, patience-trying transition period, because what you're eating is *not* diet food. It's healthful food raised to such culinary heights that if you're not aware it's low in calories and in fats/saturated fats, and devoid of added sugar and salt, you would never guess. Before my haute cuisine of health became famous, our guests never knew they were eating Diet for Life food until I told them—always *after* they had raved about the meal. My recipes lock out taste deprivation.

We continue to prove it by playing a game with our dinner guests, although they don't know they're playing. We place a salt shaker on the table. If any guest uses it, we lose. We've never lost.

How to Stay at Your Ideal Weight for the Rest of Your Life

In a famous experiment, 100 overweight people were placed on a diet under rigorous, medically supervised clinical conditions. All lost weight. But two years after the treatment, only two of those 100 were able to retain their weight loss.

If you can't keep it off, taking it off is worthless.

To keep your weight off, you need a maintenance diet—a diet that will supply you with just enough calories to hold your weight steady. A maintenance diet is a calorie-restricted diet; go over your daily caloric allowance, and you'll gain weight. You can only stay on a calorie-restricted diet for the rest of your life if it's so irresistibly delicious that it nullifies the temptation to go on a binge or stray. The Diet for Life, calorie-adjusted to meet your weight-maintenance needs, is such a diet. (To up calories, see guidelines on page 70.)

Here's how to determine:

YOUR DAILY CALORIC ALLOWANCE
FOR MAINTAINING IDEAL WEIGHT
AT ANY AGE

IDEAL WEIGHT	AGE		
Men	25–44	45–59	60 and over
110	2,300(13.5)	2,050(15)	1,750(16.5)
120	2,400(10)	2,200(17.5)	1,850(25)
130	2,550(12.5)	2,300(17.5)	1,950(22.5)
140	2,700(12.5)	2,450(20)	2,050(27.5)
150	2,850(15)	2,550(20)	2,150(25)
160	3,000(15)	2,700(22.5)	2,250(3)
170	3,100(15)	2,800(22.5)	2,350(30)
180	3,250(15)	2,950(25)	2,450(35)
190	3,400(19)	3,050(27.5)	2,600(37.5)
Women			
90	1,600(5)	1,500(12.5)	1,250(20)
100	1,750(7.5)	1,600(12.5)	1,350(17.5)
110	1,900(10)	1,700(12.5)	1,450(15)
120	2,000(10)	1,800(15)	1,500(20)
130	2,100(10)	1,900(15)	1,600(20)
140	2,250(10)	2,050(17.5)	1,700(25)
150	2,350(10)	2,150(17.5)	1,800(25)
160	2,500(12.5)	2,250(17.5)	1,900(22.5)

HOW TO USE THIS CHART *

1. Find the ideal weight nearest yours. If your ideal weight ends in 5, the ideal weight nearest yours is the lower weight.
2. Find the corresponding numerals in the column under your age group.
3. Multiply the figure in parentheses by the difference between your age and the lowest age in your age group.
4. Subtract the result from the larger figure.
5. Example: you're a 35-year-old woman whose ideal weight is 125:
   a. The ideal weight nearest yours is 120.
   b. The corresponding numerals in your age-group column are 2,000(10). See box on chart.
   c. The difference between your age (35) and the lowest age in your age group (25) is 10. Multiplying that by the figure in parentheses gives you 100 (10 × 10).
   d. 2,000 minus 100 = 1,900, which is your daily caloric allowance for maintaining your ideal weight of 125 at age 35.

---

* This chart has been compiled from U.S. Department of Agriculture statistics.

As you can see from the chart, the amount of calories you need to maintain your ideal weight decreases as you grow older. If you continue to consume the same amount of calories year after year, you'll gain weight. (This is true whether you're at ideal weight or not. That's why men and women in their 40s, who never ate more over the years than they did in their teens, have middle-age spread.)

So, each year use the chart to figure out your daily caloric allowance for maintaining ideal weight, and cut your daily caloric intake accordingly. To do so, use one or more of the following methods:

1. Eliminate some snacks.
2. Serve meals with fewer courses.
3. Decrease the size of servings.
4. Substitute lower-calorie dishes than those presently on your menus. [Be sure they're Diet for Life dishes, which you'll find in this book, and in *The Dieter's Gourmet Cookbook,* or which you'll create yourself (see Chapter 8).]

15 DON'Ts to Help You Stay on Any Diet— Reducing or Maintenance

Fat-gaining habits, both at the table and away from it, can wreck any diet, no matter how delectable. Follow the advice of these DON'T's, and you can break those habits. We did.

1. DON'T *chew gum.* Gum-chewing stimulates the salivary glands, and that can make you feel hungry even if you just have eaten a meal. If you're one of those overweight people who eats whenever you're nervous, consider this: contrary to what most people think, gum-chewing doesn't calm you down; it makes you more nervous. Sugarless gum is not an antidote to weight gain from gum-chewing. The small amount of sugar calories in regular gum won't put an ounce on you. It's the act of chewing, when you shouldn't be, that makes you want to eat when you shouldn't eat—that puts on all those pounds that you shouldn't have.

2. DON'T *drink carbonated beverages during a meal.* And that includes—heresy!—Perrier-with-lime. The carbon dioxide gas bloats you and gives you that filled-up feeling which often prevents you from finishing your food. Isn't that good because you eat less? No! It's bad because you don't enjoy what you eat; and—more important—two hours or so later, you get so hungry you ravage your refrigerator.

3. DON'T *eat rapidly.* It's the amount of food in the blood, not in the stomach, that triggers the STOP! signal when you've had enough to satisfy your body's needs. But it takes time for your food to digest and pass into the blood. Speed-eat, and you can swallow all the food your body needs before it can get into the blood and trigger the STOP! signal. Result: you go on eating. If you're as fast as some

speed-eaters, you can down the equivalent of two meals, or even three, before the STOP! signal tells you you're no longer hungry. Eating rapidly means eating more. Eating slowly means eating less—and tasting more.

4. DON'T *eat standing up*. Stand-up eaters are speed-eaters. Even if you're eating alone at home, set a table—flatware, napery, dinnerware, the works—and enjoy as leisurely a repast as if you were dining in a three-star restaurant. If you're serving your impatient family ("Ma! I gotta get to school!"), don't take *your* food on the run. Instead, plan your meal schedule so everybody can sit down at the table and be relaxed—especially you.

5. DON'T *serve your entire meal at one time*. Ever wonder why you get through those aircraft meals so fast? Served together, a three-course meal looks like a one-course meal, and you gobble it up as if it were. You're finished long before the STOP! sign flashes on, and you want more. That's one reason why most passengers feel unsatisfied after dining on a plane.

Serve your meals course by course, with a short time-out between all courses up to the entrée, and a long time-out (up to 30 minutes) between the entrée and the dessert. That gives the food ample time to get into the bloodstream. When you finally get to the dessert, the STOP! sign is about to go on and you'll never be tempted to reach for that second slice of pie.

6. DON'T *serve family style*. You'll not only eat faster, but you'll eat larger portions, and more portions. Serve restaurant style. It will cut down on your calories—and your food bills.

7. DON'T *eat all over the house*. Eat only at the dining table. That rules out eating in front of the TV, in bed, in your reading armchair, or anyplace else where you could snack yourself into overweight.

8. DON'T *go shopping for food on an empty stomach*. When hunger is the spur, you'll buy much more than you actually need, especially quick-foods like sweets, snacks, and TV dinners. Keep extra food out of your home. Out of sight is out of mouth.

9. DON'T *go shopping for food without a shopping list*. The list will help guide you past the lures of supermarket supermerchandising, and help stifle impulse buying. Make sure the list is made up only of Diet for Life favored ingredients (Chapter 9).

10. DON'T *skip breakfast*. It's the most important meal of the day. Reject food in the morning, and it will be reflected adversely in your mood, your energy, and your brain power. Worse, from the dieting point of view: you'll be tempted at coffee-break time, and ravenous by lunch. Breakfast-skippers are luncheon-overeaters, and spend distressing afternoons fighting somnolence, distention, and stupor.

11. DON'T *skip lunch*. Skipping lunch is another silly trick to

save calories. You eventually arrive at the dinner table ready to eat anything in sight, and do, usually at high speed. What's more, if you're a lunch-skipper, by mid-afternoon your blood sugar will be down, and so will you.

12. DON'T *eat on an irregular timetable.* On an irregular eating schedule, you either eat when your body doesn't need all that food, or you don't eat until your hunger pangs grow so strong that you speed-eat, consuming more than you should. A regular eating schedule conditions your body to operate on just so much food at such-and-such times. Set up a convenient eating timetable, and stick to it.

13. DON'T *cheat when you weigh yourself.* Your body weight fluctuates during the course of every 24 hours. You're at your heaviest after dinner, and at your lightest before breakfast. Weigh yourself after dinner and then the next day before breakfast, and you've miraculously lost two pounds or more. Be honest, and weigh yourself at the same time every day (before breakfast will make you feel best).

Some bathroom scales have quirks, and register lighter on some places on the floor than on others. Don't take a cheap weight loss by moving your scale around. Keep your scale in one place. And don't knock off a pound or so by getting on the scale when it registers under zero. Adjust your scale to zero before you weigh yourself.

Most important: don't weigh yourself with your clothes on. The weight of your clothes varies, and all you have to do to shed pounds is switch to a lighter outfit. Even if you wear the same clothes every day (a uniform or work clothes, for example), their weight will vary because they pick up moisture from the air. On a dry day you'll weigh less than on a humid one. Weigh yourself without clothes, and get the naked truth!

14. DON'T *think of yourself as a fat person.* Think of yourself as slim, energetic, younger looking. Then when you're tempted to stray from your healthful eating program, flash that picture in your mind. The image that you have of yourself is the image that you become. You won't stray.

And, above all—

15. DON'T *think of yourself as being on a diet.* There's nobody on a diet who doesn't desire to cheat, and desire too often becomes reality. But you're not on a diet. Remember: the Diet for Life is an eating program for slimming down healthfully and staying slim permanently while expanding the joys of the table.

You'll find basic menus and recipes for that program in the following chapters.

6

Three Weeks of Gourmet Reducing Menus

Say hello to these menus and say good-bye to bland health food forever. Read over the menus as if you were sitting down in a brand-new three-star restaurant with a fabulous cuisine you've never tasted before. The menus will be your passport to a new style of cooking, and to a cornucopia of new flavors.

What's marvelous about these menus is you don't have to go to a three-star restaurant to enjoy them. They were created to be made in a home kitchen like yours, because the only way you can enjoy delicious, healthful foods for the rest of your life is to cook them yourself. Cooking is a creative act—one of the greatest joys you'll ever experience. And an even greater joy is serving what you've created to someone you love. ("But I go to work five days a week. What about lunch?" You'll find a wholesome answer on page 90.)

How to Use the Menus

It is imperative that you read these instructions before you refer to the menus and to the recipes.

A numeral in parentheses before a menu item indicates that I've provided a recipe for it. The recipes are arranged numerically in the next chapter.

Example: On Monday of the first week, you will have for dinner:

(4) Lobster Taste-Alike (Sautéed Tile Fish)

To find the recipe, turn to (4) in the next chapter.

In addition, you'll find unnumbered recipes for My Ketchup and

All-Round Sauce on pages 195–196; and beginning on page 183, you'll find recipes for three kinds of bread, an all-purpose stock, three kinds of salad dressing, and a basic recipe for steaming vegetables.

You don't have to prepare new dishes every day. It's likely that you'll come across several dishes with which you'll fall madly in love, and you'll want to repeat them. By all means, do so. For example: the Diet for Life weekly dinner plan calls for meat, fish, and poultry each twice a week on alternate days. If you like, repeat the meat dish, or the fish dish, or the poultry dish. You can use vegetables and other dishes more than once, as well.

But fair warning: once you try one of my new haute cuisine of health dishes, you'll want to try them all. And here's a wonderful surprise: they're amazingly simple to prepare, even if you've never cooked before.

Daily menus add up to about 1,250 calories. You've learned how to adjust the amount to your specific dieting needs (pages 74 and 75). If you like, you can mix and match recipes from any of the three weeks to create new daily menus to satisfy your taste preferences— provided you stay within your allotted calories, and don't eat either meat, fish, or poultry for dinner more than twice a week on alternating days.

You can make the following substitutions in the menus:

- For each serving of fruit:
  ½ grapefruit
  4 stewed or raw prunes
  ¼ cup prune whip
  ½ cup berries in season
  ½ cup homemade applesauce
  ½ cup pineapple chunks in their own juice

- Any soup for any other

- Lettuce and tomatoes for any salad

- Any marinade for any other

- A baked, medium-sized white or a small sweet potato for any of my potato recipes

When the menu calls for cottage cheese, use only dry-curd cottage cheese, no salt added, ½% milkfat. It's available in supermarkets.

When the menu calls for salad dressing, use mine only, allowing up to two tablespoons per serving.

And here's a marvelous suprise. When you're losing weight on the Diet for Life—

You Can Snack

You can eat the following recommended portions of low-calorie food once a day. That limiting word, if you slipped over it, is *once*.

- 1 Puffed Wheat Cookie (page 138) or Apple-Oatmeal Cookie (see *The Dieter's Gourmet Cookbook*)
- 14 spoon-sized shredded-wheat biscuits
- ½ cup freshly made popcorn, no salt or butter added
- 2–3 tablespoons dry-curd cottage cheese (½% milkfat) on a saltless brown rice or wheat wafer, sprinkled with freshly minced dill or grated orange rind
- 1 tablespoon raisins and 1 whole walnut
- 4 California dates
- 2 dried prunes
- ½ banana
- 1 rib celery
- 1 small carrot
- 6 radishes
- ½ small cucumber
- Several sprigs fresh watercress or arrugula
- 4 flowerettes raw or blanched broccoli
- ½ small endive
- 4 ounces apple juice, no sugar added
- 4 ounces tomato juice, no salt added

On a weight-maintenance diet, you can snack twice a day, and you can increase portions to comply with your daily caloric allowance. And you can even treat yourself to a milk shake (page 140), but no more than one a day.

And a big plus—on both the reducing and the maintenance diets, begin your day with the best snack of all: our energy-boosting vitamin cocktail (pages 259 and 266).

Major Dinner Recipes

MEAT

FIRST WEEK: Sweet Veal Loaf
Sautéed Steak with Wine

SECOND WEEK: Broiled Curried Veal Chops
Skillet Meat Balls with Savory Sauce

THIRD WEEK: Marinated Beef with Vegetables
Chili Pork Chops

FISH

FIRST WEEK: Lobster Taste-Alike (Sautéed Tile Fish)
Quick and Fantastic Scrod

SECOND WEEK: Striped Bass Steaks with Barbeque Sauce
Gray Sole Paupiettes

THIRD WEEK: Succulent Broiled Flounder
Crisp and Moist Fillet of Lemon Sole

CHICKEN

FIRST WEEK: Broiled Herbed Chicken
Quick and Easy Sautéed Chicken Breasts

SECOND WEEK: Roast Orange Chicken
Simple Lemon Curry Chicken

THIRD WEEK: Chicken with Yams
Stuffed Cornish Hens with Grape Sauce

VEGETARIAN SUNDAY DINNERS

FIRST WEEK: Pasta with Curried Tomato Sauce

SECOND WEEK: Mushroom and Rice Patties

THIRD WEEK: Baked Stuffed Eggplant

Your Gourmet Reducing Menus: First Week

Monday

BREAKFAST:
Whole orange
(1) Spiced Oatmeal
(2) 3 ounces non-fat milk, or French Coffee

LUNCH:
(3) Thick Minestrone Soup
1 slice bread
Mixed green salad with one of my salad dressings
1 serving fresh fruit

DINNER
1 cup tomato juice, no salt added
(4) Lobster Taste-Alike (Tile Fish)
Steamed green beans
1 slice bread
(5) Hawaiian Applesauce

Tuesday

BREAKFAST:
(6) ½ grapefruit, raw or broiled, sprinkled with 1 teaspoon toasted
wheat germ, no sugar added
(7) Oriental Omelette, or poached egg on toast
1 slice bread
(2) Herb mint tea, or French Coffee

LUNCH:
(8) Cottage Cheese Sundae
1 slice bread
3 ounces non-fat milk

DINNER: (9)   Broiled Herbed Chicken
             (10)   Fresh Asparagus Almondine
                    Scallions, crisp watercress, and sliced tomato
                    1 serving fresh fruit

Wednesday
BREAKFAST: ½ cup fresh orange juice, or whole orange
                    Puffed wheat, no sugar or salt added, with ½ cup berries in
                        season, or ½ banana
                    1 cup non-fat milk

LUNCH: (11)   Tuna Supreme
                    1 slice bread
                    ½ small cucumber, sliced
                    Small sliced tomato
                    Several sprigs crisp watercress
                    3 ounces non-fat milk

DINNER: (12)   Sweet Veal Loaf
                    Mixed green salad with one of my salad dressings
                    Small baked sweet potato
                    1 serving fresh fruit

Thursday
BREAKFAST: Wedge of melon in season
                    1 cake shredded wheat sprinkled with 1 teaspoon toasted
                        wheat germ, no sugar added
                    1 medium banana
                    1 cup non-fat milk

LUNCH: (13)   Special Spanish Rice
                    Crisp watercress sprigs and scallions
                    1 cup apple juice, no sugar added

DINNER: (14)   Quick and Fantastic Scrod
             (15)   Dilled Mashed Potatoes
                    1 slice bread
                    Steamed carrots
                    ½ cup pineapple chunks in their own juice

Friday
BREAKFAST: Whole orange
             (16)   Cream of Wheat, New Style
              (2)   3 ounces non-fat milk, or French Coffee

LUNCH: (17)   Mushroom and Barley Soup
                    1 slice bread
                    1 serving fresh fruit

DINNER: (18) Quick and Easy Sautéed Chicken Breasts
           (19) Baked Sweet Rice
                Crudités: colorfully arranged raw vegetables
           (5) Hawaiian Applesauce

Saturday
BREAKFAST: (20) Sweet Baked Apples
                1 slice toast with cottage cheese (½% milkfat)
           (2) 3 ounces non-fat milk, or French Coffee

LUNCH: (21) Curried Mushrooms on Toast
                ½ cup pineapple chunks in their own juice

DINNER: (22) Sautéed Steak with Wine
           (23) Skillet-Browned Potatoes
                Small mixed green salad with 2 teaspoons of one of my salad
                   dressings
           (24) Poached Pears in Calvados with Spiced Meringue Topping

Sunday
BREAKFAST: ½ cup orange juice, or whole orange
           (25) Spiced Griddle Cakes, or poached egg on toast
           (2) 3 ounces non-fat milk, or French Coffee

LUNCH: (26) Sautéed Chinese-Style Vegetables and Fruit
           (27) Fluffy and Delicious Boiled Rice
                Herb mint tea

DINNER: (28) Pasta with Curried Tomato Sauce
                Small mixed green salad with 2 teaspoons of one of my salad
                   dressings
                ½ cup pineapple chunks in their own juice
           (29) Tangy Buckwheat Brownies

Your Gourmet Reducing Menus: Second Week

Monday
BREAKFAST: (6) ½ grapefruit, raw or broiled, sprinkled with 1 teaspoon toasted
                  wheat germ, no sugar added
           (30) Jiffy Orange Muffins
           (2) 3 ounces non-fat milk, or French Coffee

LUNCH: (31) One-Step Chilled Fruit Soup
                1 slice bread
                Mixed green salad with one of my salad dressings

DINNER: (32) Roast Orange Chicken
                Small baked sweet potato
           (33) Stir-Fried Zucchini with Apples
                ½ cup berries or grapes in season

Tuesday

BREAKFAST: (34) Sweet Stewed Prunes
⅔ cup spoon-sized shredded wheat sprinkled with 1 teaspoon toasted wheat germ, no sugar added, or poached egg on toast
1 cup non-fat milk

LUNCH: Chicken sandwich with watercress and tomato
1 serving fresh fruit

DINNER: 1 cup tomato juice, no salt added
(35) Striped Bass Steaks with Barbeque Sauce
(36) Watercress and Endive Salad with one of my salad dressings
(37) 2 Puffed Wheat Cookies

Wednesday

BREAKFAST: Wedge of melon in season, or ½ cup berries
(1) Spiced Oatmeal sprinkled with 1 teaspoon toasted wheat germ, no sugar added
1 slice toast with 1 teaspoon honey
(2) 3 ounces non-fat milk, or French Coffee

LUNCH: (38) Boston Salad with any variation
1 slice bread
(39) Frothy Fruit Milk Shake

DINNER: (40) Broiled Curried Veal Chops
(41) Quick-Cooking Kasha (Buckwheat Groats)
Steamed green beans
½ cup pineapple chunks in their own juice
(37) 2 Puffed Wheat Cookies

Thursday

BREAKFAST: Whole orange
(42) Sweet French Toast
Herb mint tea

LUNCH: (43) Chilled Baby Bean Salad
2 brown rice or wheat wafers, crisped
(39) Frothy Fruit Milk Shake

DINNER: (44) Simple Lemon Curry Chicken
Small baked sweet potato
Mixed green salad with one of my salad dressings
(45) Apple Whip

Friday

BREAKFAST: (46) Prune Whip
(47) Apple Pancakes
Herb mint tea

LUNCH   Sliced chicken served on a bed of lettuce garnished with watercress, scallions, and tomatoes
2 brown rice or wheat wafers, crisped
1 cup tomato juice, no salt added

DINNER: (48)   Gray Sole Paupiettes
(49)   Gingered Rice and Carrots
(50)   Broiled Tomatoes
1 serving fresh fruit

Saturday
BREAKFAST: (20)   Sweet Baked Apple
1 slice toast with cottage cheese (½% milkfat)
(2)   3 ounces non-fat milk, or French Coffee

LUNCH: (17)   Mushroom and Barley Soup
1 slice bread
1 serving fresh fruit

DINNER: (51)   Skillet Meatballs with Savory Sauce
(52)   Minted Peas
Small baked sweet potato
(53)   Apple Whip Sherbet

Sunday
BREAKFAST: Whole orange
1 cake shredded wheat sprinkled with 1 teaspoon toasted
wheat germ, no sugar added, or poached egg on toast
1 cup non-fat milk

LUNCH: (54)   Creamy Egg Salad Sandwich with lettuce and tomatoes
1 serving fresh fruit
(29)   1 Tangy Buckwheat Brownie

DINNER: 1 cup tomato juice, no salt added
(55)   Caraway Cheese Dip with crisped brown rice wafers
(56)   Mushroom and Rice Patties
Steamed carrots sprinkled with fresh dill and minced shallots
(57)   Pineapple-Banana Mousse

Your Gourmet Reducing Menus: Third Week

Monday
BREAKFAST: ½ cup orange juice
(30)   Jiffy Orange Muffins with cottage cheese (½% milkfat)
(2)   3 ounces non-fat milk, or French Coffee

LUNCH: (58)   Steamed Artichokes with Vinaigrette Dressing
1 slice bread
1 serving fresh fruit

DINNER: (59) Succulent Broiled Flounder
            (23) Baked potato, or Skillet-Browned Potatoes
                  Crudités: artfully arranged raw vegetables
            (60) One-Bowl Mystery Cake

Tuesday
BREAKFAST: Whole orange
                  ⅔ cup spoon-sized shredded wheat sprinkled with 1 teaspoon
                  toasted wheat germ, no sugar added, or poached egg on
                  toast
                  1 cup non-fat milk

LUNCH: (61) Fruit Chiffon Mold
                  1 slice bread, or ½ plain matzoh
                  1 cup apple juice, no sugar added
            (29) 1 Tangy Buckwheat Brownie

DINNER: (17) Mushroom and Barley Soup
            (62) Chicken with Yams
            (63) Tart Savory Cabbage
                  ½ cup pineapple chunks in their own juice

Wednesday
BREAKFAST: (6) ½ grapefruit, raw or broiled
             (1) Spiced Oatmeal
             (2) 3 ounces non-fat milk, or French Coffee

LUNCH: (64) Crunchy Chicken Salad
                  1 cup tomato juice, no salt added
                  Herb mint tea

DINNER: (65) Marinated Beef with Vegetables
            (27) Fluffy and Delicious Boiled Rice
                  Small mixed green salad with 2 teaspoons of one of my salad
                     dressings
            (66) Mocha Sponge

Thursday
BREAKFAST: Wedge of melon, or ½ cup berries in season
            (42) Sweet French Toast with 2 teaspoons honey
             (2) Herb mint tea, or French Coffee

LUNCH: (67) Curried Tomato-Pea Soup
                  1 slice bread
                  1 serving fresh fruit

DINNER: 1 cup tomato juice, no salt added
            (68) Crisp and Moist Fillet of Lemon Sole
                  Steamed green beans
            (15) Dilled Mashed Potatoes
            (39) Frothy Fruit Milk Shake
            (37) 2 Puffed Wheat Cookies

Friday

BREAKFAST: (34) Sweet Stewed Prunes
 (16) Cream of Wheat, New Style
 (2) 3 ounces non-fat milk, or French Coffee

LUNCH Brisling sardines, no salt added, packed in spring water
 1 small tomato
 Several watercress sprigs
 1 slice bread
 ½ cup apple juice, no sugar added

DINNER: (69) Stuffed Cornish Hens with Grape Sauce
 Steamed Brussels sprouts
 (70) Grape Sherbet
 (37) 2 Puffed Wheat Cookies

Saturday

BREAKFAST: (20) Sweet Baked Apple sprinkled with 1 teaspoon toasted wheat
 germ, no sugar added
 1 slice toast with 1 teaspoon flavorful honey
 (2) 3 ounces non-fat milk, or French Coffee

LUNCH: (8) Cottage Cheese Sundae
 2 brown rice or wheat wafers, crisped
 Herb mint tea

DINNER: (71) Chili Pork Chops
 (72) Sweet Potato-Apple Mélange
 ½ cup pineapple chunks in their own juice

Sunday

BREAKFAST: Whole orange
 (47) Apple Pancakes
 (2) 3 ounces non-fat milk, or French Coffee

LUNCH: (17) Mushroom and Barley Soup
 1 slice bread
 2 tablespoons raisins and 2 walnuts

DINNER: (73) Baked Stuffed Eggplant
 Steamed carrots
 (74) Buttermilk Coleslaw
 (75) Fallen Angel Food Cake with Berry Topping

The Working Dieter's Guide to Lunchtime

Because of the soaring costs of eating lunches out, some companies have installed low-cost cafeterias on their premises; and others
provide pleasantly decorated and furnished lunchrooms, equipped

with refrigerators, sink, and stove, for those who prefer to eat their own food.

If there is a low-cost cafeteria at your disposal, you can enjoy salads, fresh fruit, and unsweetened fruit juices daily. But a low-cost cafeteria has all the perils of any eatery (including a health-food restaurant)—hidden quantities of sugar, salt, and fat in most of the food—so don't let those attractive counter displays entice you. Besides, a low-cost cafeteria has a peril all its own: the food is so cheap, you tend to overeat.

The only practical way to have varied, tasty lunches that satisfy low-caloric and high nutritional standards is to brown-paper-bag it. The cost is even lower than the low-cost cafeteria's; and in these days of rampant inflation, it's chic to save.

Some hints:

1. Buy a wide-mouthed Thermos that will hold an ample portion of hot or cold soup, cottage cheese, tuna salad, sliced cold chicken or turkey, and sliced cold vegetables.

2. To keep food very hot, wash out the Thermos, then fill it with hot (not boiling) water, and let stand, covered, for five minutes. Pour out the water. Then fill with well-heated soup or any hot food. Cover tightly.

3. To keep foods very cold, fill the Thermos with cold water, and let stand for five minutes. Pour out the water. Then fill with cold soup or any other food you wish to keep cold. Your salad greens will emerge refreshingly cool and crisp at lunchtime.

4. If you have a yen for a sandwich at lunch, you can use your Thermos to make up one fresh. Here's what you do: prepare the Thermos as you would for cold food. Add any combination of fillers, like cold sliced meat, fish, chicken, crisp lettuce leaves, cucumbers, and tomatoes. Cover tightly. Wrap sliced bread in wax paper. Just before eating, unwrap paper, open Thermos, and lay filling on bread.

Try eating your sandwich open-faced. It's like having two sandwiches instead of one; eating takes longer, and you get a more "satisfied" feeling.

And talking of open-faced sandwiches, did you know that, in Denmark, almost everybody eats them for lunch? And most workers take them from home and eat them where they work. When you brown-paper-bag it, it's comforting to know millions of other people are doing the same thing.

It takes only five minutes or so in the morning to prepare your lunch, and the dividends are greater than just dollars saved. You'll escape the hustle and bustle of eating out. You'll have time to relax. And, above all, you'll be staying on your Diet for Life program—and that should give you a sense of accomplishment and a feeling of good health.

Once you've achieved your ideal weight, you can most certainly eat lunch out once a week. But remember: no salty cold cuts and cheeses, and *never, never* pickles or relishes. Roast beef or turkey are good bets; but if you're having them in a sandwich, stay away from rolls; they're more caloric and salty than sliced bread. Adhere to these restrictions; then, once a month, treat yourself to one of your favorite desserts. It will have virtually no effect on your weight.

While you're on the reducing diet or the maintenance diet, spin off on the lunch dishes to create a varied array of portable feasts. That will help make lunchtime—as it should be—fun time.

7

115 *New* Gourmet Recipes and Variations for Dieters

Following each recipe, you'll find this line:

CAL	F	P:S	SOD	CAR	CHO

CAL stands for food energy in calories; F for fat in grams; P:S for the ratio of polyunsaturated fats to saturated fats; SOD for sodium in milligrams; CAR for carbohydrates in grams; and CHO for cholesterol in milligrams. Figures under each heading represent quantities per serving. They have been calculated mainly from data on the composition of foods made available by the Agricultural Research Service of the United States Department of Agriculture. Figures have been rounded out to the nearest .5, except for P's which are given to the nearest tenth. When a quantity is less than .25, it is regarded as 0, except when it's a P quantity, in which case less than .25 is designated as "trace." Because no two equal-amount samples of the same kind of food are certain to have exactly the same nutritional values, the numerals following each recipe should be considered approximations, albeit close ones.

(1) Spiced Oatmeal

    2 tablespoons apple juice, no sugar added
    ⅔ cup water
    ⅓ cup old-fashioned rolled oats
    3 dashes ground ginger
    2 dashes ground cloves
      Cinnamon to taste

For a smooth-textured cereal:
1. Combine all ingredients except cinnamon in small saucepan. Bring to boil. Turn heat down, and gently simmer for 8-10 minutes, stirring often.
2. Cover and let stand for 2 minutes.
3. Pour into cereal bowl, sprinkle with cinnamon, and serve.

For a thicker, more chunky cereal:
1. Combine apple juice, water, cloves, and ginger in small saucepan. Bring to boil. Add oatmeal and stir. Turn heat down and gently simmer for 8-10 minutes, stirring often.
2. Cover and let stand for 2 minutes.
3. Pour into cereal bowl, sprinkle with cinnamon, and serve.

YIELD: Serves 1

VARIATION: Sprinkle cooked cereal with one tablespoon toasted wheat germ, no sugar added.

CAL	F	P:S	SOD	CAR	CHO
120	2	2:1	10	20	0
With wheat germ:					
133	3	2.5:1	10	23	0

(2) French Coffee

⅓ cup equal parts water and apple juice combined, no sugar added
½ teaspoon decaffeinated coffee
1 teaspoon coffee substitute
⅛ teaspoon ground cinnamon
½ cup non-fat liquid milk

1. Combine first four ingredients in small saucepan and bring to boil, stirring to blend.
2. Turn down heat. Add milk and bring to simmering point. Serve.

YIELD: Serves 1

CAL	F	P:S	SOD	CAR	CHO
80	0	—	45	11	3.5

(3) Thick Minestrone Soup

½ cup white beans
2 cups stock (page 187)
3 cups water
2 tablespoons corn oil
3 cloves garlic, minced
2 medium onions, minced
1 large rib celery, minced
3 large fresh mushrooms, coarsely chopped
½ cup thinly sliced cabbage
2 tablespoons wine vinegar
1 8¼-ounce can tomatoes, no salt added
2½ tablespoons tomato paste, no salt added
½ cup diced carrots
5 whole cloves
6 dashes cayenne pepper
1¼ teaspoons combined dried sage and rosemary
    leaves, crushed
    Large bouquet garni
½ cup whole-wheat macaroni
1 cup diced zucchini (optional)

1. Soak beans overnight in water to cover. Drain. Transfer to waterless cooker or heavy-bottomed saucepan. Add one cup stock and 2 cups water. Cover and cook until tender.

2. Heat oil in large non-stick skillet until hot. Sauté garlic, onions, celery, and mushrooms until wilted.

3. Add cabbage and sauté for 3-4 minutes until volume of cabbage shrinks.

4. Add vinegar and cook 1 minute.

5. Pour sautéed mixture into cooked beans. Add balance of stock, water, tomatoes, tomato paste, carrots, cloves, cayenne, herbs, and bouquet garni. Bring to simmering point. Partially cover and simmer for 20 minutes.

6. Add macaroni and optional zucchini, partially cover, and simmer for 15 minutes. Turn off heat. Let soup stand for 45 minutes. Reheat just before serving.

YIELD: Serves 6 as main course; serves 10 as first course

VARIATION: Grated Sap Sago cheese, ½ teaspoon per serving, may be sprinkled on top of soup. For other low-fat cheeses, see page 249.

CAL	F	P:S	SOD	CAR	CHO
Serves 6:					
171	5	4.5:1	52	22.5	0
Serves 10:					
102.5	3	4.5:1	32	13.5	0
With zucchini, serves 6:					
176	5	4.5:1	52	23	0
With zucchini, serves 10:					
105.5	0	4.5:1	32	14	0
With Sap Sago:					
No appreciable difference					

(4) Lobster Taste-Alike
(Sautéed Tile Fish)

    4   fresh tile fish fillets, 1½ pounds
    ½   teaspoon each ground ginger and crushed sweet
        basil leaves
    6   dashes cayenne pepper
    1   tablespoon corn oil
    2   large cloves garlic, finely minced
    2   shallots, finely minced
    1   small rib celery, finely minced
    1   small onion, finely minced
    1   tablespoon finely minced green pepper
    ⅓   cup dry vermouth
        Lemon wedges

1. Wash fish and pat dry with paper toweling. Sprinkle on both sides with equal amounts of ginger, basil, and cayenne.

2. Heat oil in non-stick skillet until hot. Add garlic, shallots, and minced vegetables. Sauté for one minute. Spread mixture evenly over skillet.

3. Lay fillets on top of mixture and sauté over medium-high heat for 5 minutes. Turn and sauté for 2 minutes.

4. Add vermouth, and cook for 3 minutes, continually spooning sauce over fish. Fish is done when it flakes easily.

5. Arrange on warm serving plates, spoon with sauce, and garnish with lemon wedges.

YIELD: Serves 4

VARIATION: Include 2 fresh mushrooms, washed, dried, trimmed, and coarsely chopped, in Step #2.

NOTE:

1. Fillet of lemon sole, gray sole, scrod, or flounder may be substituted for tile fish.

2. Cooking time will vary with thickness of fish.

3. Non-stick skillets do not withstand high heat, so cooking time is longer than with conventional cookware.

CAL	F	P:S	SOD	CAR	CHO
193	4.5	3.6:1	32.5	4.9	94.5

Variation:
No appreciable difference
With scrod:

194	3.9	3.7:1	34.5	5	94.5

With flounder or sole:
No appreciable difference

(5) Hawaiian Applesauce

4 crisp sweet apples, cored and sliced
⅓ cup unsweetened pineapple juice
4 whole cloves
4 dashes ground allspice
½ teaspoon ground cinnamon
3 dashes ground nutmeg
1 slice orange, including skin

1. Combine all ingredients in heavy-bottomed pot or waterless cooker. Bring to simmering point. Cover and simmer for 10 minutes. Partially uncover, and let cool in pot. Discard orange slice.
2. Pour into food mill and purée.

YIELD: Serves 4 with one leftover portion

NOTE: Combine Cortland and Delicious, and/or Winesap apples for excellent flavor and texture.

CAL	F	P:S	SOD	CAR	CHO
68	0	—	4	2	0

(6) Broiled Grapefruit

    1   sweet grapefruit, cut in half
    ¼ cup apple juice, no sugar added
    ¼ teaspoon ground cinnamon
    4 dashes ground nutmeg

1. Cut flesh of grapefruit into segments, separate from skin, and leave in shell.

2. Place halves in shallow baking dish. Pour equal amounts of apple juice over each half. Sprinkle with cinnamon and nutmeg.

3. Broil 2″ from heat for 10-12 minutes. Serve hot.

YIELD: Serves 2

NOTE: If grapefruit is not sweet enough for your taste, spoon ½ teaspoon flavorful honey over each half before broiling.

CAL	F	P:S	SOD	CAR	CHO
45	0	—	3	4	0
With honey:					
50	0	—	3	4.5	0

(7) Oriental Omelette

For the filling:

    2 teaspoons corn oil
    1 small onion, thinly sliced
    1 whole scallion, diagonally cut into ½″ pieces
    1 small clove garlic, minced
    1 cake tofu (bean curd) cut 3″ square, pat dry with paper toweling, and cut into 12 cubes
    2 dashes cayenne pepper
    ¼ teaspoon ground ginger
    ¼ teaspoon low-sodium soy sauce (available in health-food stores)

For the eggs:

    ¼ teaspoon corn oil
    4 egg whites
    2 dashes cayenne pepper
    4 dashes ground ginger

1. Prepare filling first. Heat oil in 8″ non-stick skillet until hot. Add onion, scallion, and garlic. Sauté for 2 minutes.

2. Add tofu. Sprinkle with cayenne, ginger, and soy sauce. Stir and cook until hot. Pour into small bowl and cover to keep warm. Wipe out skillet.

3. Drop egg whites into small bowl together with cayenne and ginger. Beat with fork until frothy.

4. Brush skillet with oil. Heat until hot but not smoking. Add eggs, tilting pan in a complete circle until eggs reach all sides of skillet. Cook until lightly browned on one side. Center should remain moist. Slide onto plate.

5. Spoon vegetable mixture over half of omelette. Flip over other side of omelette. Cut in half and serve.

YIELD: Serves 2

VARIATION: For a chili-flavored omelette, substitute ¼ teaspoon chili con carne seasoning (no salt or pepper added) for low-sodium soy sauce.

CAL	F	P:S	SOD	CAR	CHO
Filling:					
139	12	4.5:1	35.5	4.5	0
Eggs:					
27	2.2	4.5:1	110	0	0
Variation:					
No appreciable difference					

(8) Cottage Cheese Sundae

2 tablespoons dry-curd cottage cheese, no salt added,
   less than ½% milkfat
1 serving fresh fruit, sliced, or ½ cup pineapple chunks
   in their own juices
2 tablespoons low-fat plain yogurt
2 whole walnuts, broken into pieces
1 tablespoon raisins
1 teaspoon toasted wheat germ, no sugar added
   Cinnamon to taste
1 teaspoon honey (optional)

1. Spoon cottage cheese into cereal bowl.
2. Add fruit and yogurt.
3. Sprinkle with raisins, wheat germ, and cinnamon.
4. Top with optional honey.

YIELD: Serves 1

VARIATION: Prepare a sauce as follows in place of plain yogurt: combine 2 tablespoons yogurt with 1 teaspoon honey, 2 dashes nutmeg, and 1 dash each cinnamon and ground cloves. Stir to blend. Pour over assembled ingredients in recipe.

CAL	F	P:S	SOD	CAR	CHO
287	11	1.5:1	140.5	40.5	2
With honey:					
292	11	1.5:1	140.5	42	2
Sauce:					
46	1	.1:1	2	21.5	2

(9) Broiled Herbed Chicken

    4   large cloves garlic, minced
    3   large shallots, minced
    2   tablespoons corn oil, plus ½ teaspoon to oil broiling
        pan
    ⅓   cup combination apple-cider vinegar and wine
        vinegar
    ½   teaspoon ground ginger
    3   dashes cayenne pepper
    2   tablespoons freshly minced parsley and dill
    ½   teaspoon each dried rosemary, sage, and thyme
        leaves, crushed
    1   3-pound broiling chicken, quartered, skinned, wing
        tips removed

1. Prepare marinade by combining first 8 ingredients in jar and shaking well.

2. Wash chicken and pat dry with paper toweling. Place in deep bowl. Pour marinade over chicken, turning to coat. Cover and refrigerate for at least 6 hours. Remove from refrigerator one hour before cooking.

3. Remove chicken from marinade, reserving marinade, and place in lightly oiled shallow broiling pan. Broil 3″ from heat for 7 minutes. Turn, spoon with marinade, and broil for 7 minutes. Continue broiling, turning, and spooning with marinade until chicken is done (about 30-35 minutes). Do not overcook. Chicken should be crispy on outside, and slightly pink near bone.

YIELD: Serves 4

CAL	F	P:S	SOD	CAR	CHO
273	13.5	2.3:1	75	4	143

(10) Fresh Asparagus Amandine

1¼ pounds fresh asparagus, well washed, tough ends removed
2 tablespoons corn oil
2 large cloves garlic, finely minced
2 shallots, finely minced
1 teaspoon apple-cider vinegar
4 dashes cayenne pepper
1 teaspoon freshly minced tarragon or basil leaves
¼ teaspoon finely grated orange rind, preferably from navel orange
1 tablespoon unblanched slivered almonds, no salt added

1. Lay asparagus flat in wide-bottomed saucepan. Add ½ cup water. Bring to simmering point. Cover and simmer for 8 minutes. (Cooking time may vary with thickness of asparagus.) Drain and place on serving dish. Cover to keep warm. Wipe out saucepan.

2. Heat oil in saucepan until hot. Add garlic and shallots and sauté until wilted but not brown.

3. Add vinegar and cook 30 seconds.

4. Remove from heat. Sprinkle with cayenne, tarragon, and orange rind. Stir quickly to blend.

5. Spoon over asparagus. Top with almonds.

YIELD: Serves 4

NOTE: Fresh herbs are particularly delicious on asparagus. If fresh tarragon or basil is not available, use minced fresh dill.

CAL	F	P:S	SOD	CAR	CHO
118	9.5	4.4:1	14.5	6.5	0

(11) Tuna Supreme

    1 6½-ounce can tuna fish, packed in water, no salt
       added
    1 tablespoon fresh lemon juice
    3 tablespoons Zesty Salad Dressing or Tomato Juice
       Dressing (pages 184–186)
    ½ rib celery, finely minced
    1 small onion, grated
    4 dashes cayenne pepper
    2 teaspoons minced fresh dill
    ½ cup fresh peas, cooked and cooled
       Boston or romaine lettuce leaves, well washed and
       patted dry
    2 tomatoes, thinly sliced
       Several sprigs crisp watercress

1. Drain water from can. Transfer tuna to small bowl. Add lemon juice and salad dressing, mashing with fork to desired consistency.
2. Stir in celery, onion, cayenne, and dill. Gently fold peas into mixture.
3. Spoon equal amounts on bed of lettuce leaves, and garnish with tomatoes and watercress.

YIELD: Serves 4

VARIATION: To make a *pâté*-like, spreadable mixture, combine first 8 ingredients in a food processer, and process to desired consistency.

CAL	F	P:S	SOD	CAR	CHO
88	4.5	2.7:1	49	8.5	17.5
Variation:					
79	4.5	2.7:1	44.5	7	17.5

(12) Sweet Veal Loaf

    1   pound lean veal, ground
    3   tablespoons matzoh crumbs
    1   crisp sweet apple, peeled, cored, and coarsely
        chopped
    1½ tablespoons combined corn oil and Italian olive oil
    1   medium onion, finely minced
    3   large cloves garlic, finely minced
    2   shallots, finely minced
    3   tablespoons finely minced green pepper
    3   large fresh mushrooms, washed, dried, trimmed,
        and coarsely chopped
    ½   teaspoon each ground allspice and ginger
    6   dashes cayenne pepper
    1   teaspoon fresh tarragon leaves, minced, or ½
        teaspoon dried tarragon leaves, crushed
    ½   teaspoon ground cinnamon
    ½   cup apple juice, no sugar added
        Several sprigs watercress

1. Combine meat with crumbs and apple, blending well.
2. Heat oil in small iron skillet until hot. Add onion, garlic, shallots, green pepper, and mushrooms. Sauté until lightly brown. Sprinkle with allspice, ginger, cayenne, and tarragon, stirring to blend.
3. Pour sautéed mixture into meat and blend. Shape into 8″ x 4″ loaf. Place in rectangular baking dish which has been lined with aluminum foil.
4. Sprinkle with cinnamon. Cover loosely with lightly oiled sheet of waxed paper. Bake in preheated 400° oven for 15 minutes. Pour off any fat that may have dripped from meat.
5. Pour ¼ cup apple juice over loaf. Return to oven, re-cover with paper, and bake 10 minutes. Pour balance of apple juice over meat, re-cover, and bake an additional 10 minutes.
6. Transfer to heated serving plate, garnish with watercress, and serve.

YIELD: Serves 4

CAL	F	P:S	SOD	CAR	CHO
257	11	1.4:1	103.5	14.5	120

(13) Special Spanish Rice

1½	tablespoons combined corn oil and Italian olive oil
1	rib celery, minced
1	medium onion, minced
2	large cloves garlic, minced
2	large shallots, minced
1	small green pepper, finely minced
1½	cups cooked rice
2	tablespoons dry vermouth
2	tablespoons tomato paste, no salt added
1	8¼-ounce can tomatoes, no salt added, chopped
¼	teaspoon each ground ginger and thyme leaves, crushed
6	dashes cayenne pepper
½	teaspoon dried marjoram leaves, crushed
2	tablespoons minced fresh dill
1	teaspoon grated Sap Sago cheese (available in gourmet and cheese shops)

1. Heat oil in large non-stick skillet until hot. Add celery, onion, garlic, shallots, and green pepper and sauté over medium-high heat until lightly browned.

2. Add rice, stirring well.

3. Add vermouth and cook for 1 minute.

4. Combine tomato paste with tomatoes and balance of ingredients. Pour over rice mixture and stir until blended and well heated. Cover and let stand for 15 minutes. Re-heat and serve piping hot.

YIELD: Serves 4

VARIATION: Reduce rice to 1 cup and add 1 cup cooked meat—chicken or turkey—to recipe.

NOTE: Fresh basil or tarragon may be substituted for dill.

CAL	F	P:S	SOD	CAR	CHO
166.5	5	2.9:1	44	23	0
With veal:					
181	6.5	2.7:1	58.5	23	25
With beef:					
180	6.5	2.7:1	62	23	20
With chicken:					
170	6.5	2.9:1	56.5	23	17
With turkey:					
177.5	6.5	2.9:1	64	23	17

(14) Quick and Fantastic Scrod

1½ pounds of fillets of scrod
1½ tablespoons fresh lime juice
¾ teaspoon dried marjoram leaves, crushed
1 large clove garlic, minced
1 large shallot, minced
⅓ cup stock (page 187)
¼ cup each dry vermouth and apple juice, no sugar added
1 bay leaf
¼ teaspoon ground ginger
½ teaspoon dry mustard
4 dashes cayenne pepper
1 tablespoon minced fresh dill
2 teaspoons arrowroot flour dissolved in 1 tablespoon water

1. Wash fish. Pat dry with paper toweling. Rub on both sides with lime juice, and sprinkle with marjoram, pressing into fish.

2. Combine balance of ingredients, except flour, in large skillet. Bring to boil. Turn down heat and simmer for 2 minutes.

3. Add fish, spooning liquid over it. Bring to simmering point. Cover, and simmer for 6 minutes. Turn fish over gently. Re-cover and simmer for 6 minutes. Discard bayleaf. Transfer fish with large slotted spatula to individual serving plates.

4. Turn up heat under skillet. Dribble in arrowroot flour mixture, stirring constantly, using only enough to slightly thicken sauce. Pour over fish and serve.

YIELD: Serves 4

CAL	F	P:S	SOD	CAR	CHO
173	1.5	.8:1	154	8	106

(15) Dilled Mashed Potatoes

    3-4 potatoes, about 1¼ pounds, peeled, cubed, and
         cooked
      1 tablespoon combined corn oil and Italian olive oil
      2 large cloves garlic, minced
      2 large shallots, minced
      2 tablespoons finely minced onion or scallion
      1 teaspoon wine vinegar
      4 dashes cayenne pepper
    1½ tablespoons minced fresh dill
      ½ tablespoon minced fresh parsley
      1 teaspoon grated Sap Sago cheese (available in
         gourmet and cheese shops)
      3 tablespoons low-fat plain yogurt

1. Mash potatoes while still warm.
2. Heat oil in non-stick skillet until hot. Add garlic, shallots, onion or scallion, and sauté until wilted. Add vinegar, and cook 30 seconds.
3. Combine potatoes with sautéed mixture, together with cayenne, dill, parsley, and cheese, blending well.
4. Stir in yogurt. Re-heat over very low flame in non-stick pan, and serve.

YIELD: Serves 4

NOTE: This dish may be prepared ahead of time, turned into 4 lightly oiled serving crocks, and baked in a pre-heated 400° oven for 20-25 minutes.

CAL	F	P:S	SOD	CAR	CHO
135.5	15	2.6:1	18	21	.5

(16) Cream of Wheat, New Style

2 tablespoons apple juice, no sugar added
1¼ cups water
2½ tablespoons cream of wheat
2 dashes ground nutmeg
3 dashes ground cinnamon
1 tablespoon toasted wheat germ, no sugar added

1. Combine apple juice and water in small saucepan. Bring to rolling boil. Sprinkle in cream of wheat, nutmeg, and cinnamon, stirring constantly.
2. Lower heat and cook for 8 minutes, stirring occasionally.
3. Pour into serving dish. Sprinkle with wheat germ and serve.

YIELD: Serves 1

CAL	F	P:S	SOD	CAR	CHO
142	0	—	11	32	0

(17) Mushroom and Barley Soup

    3   teaspoons corn oil
    1   small onion, minced
    3   cloves garlic, minced
    1   rib celery, minced
    1   leek, white part only, well washed and minced
    ¼   pound lean beef, cut into small cubes, patted dry
    1   teaspoon each apple-cider vinegar and wine
        vinegar
    1   small carrot, peeled and diced
    ½   ounce imported dry, dark mushrooms, soaked until
        soft, squeezed dry, and minced
    ¼   cup medium barley, washed and drained
    ½   cup stock (page 187)
    2½ cups water
    2   teaspoons tomato paste, no salt added
    ½   teaspoon each dried thyme and rosemary leaves,
        crushed
    4   dashes cayenne pepper
        Bouquet garni

1. Heat 2 teaspoons oil in non-stick skillet until hot. Add onion, garlic, celery, and leek and sauté for 2 minutes. Push mixture to side of skillet.

2. Add meat and sauté until lightly browned on all sides. Stir meat into minced mixture.

3. Add vinegars and cook for one minute.

4. Pour into medium-sized kettle. Add balance of ingredients. Bring to simmering point, partially cover, and simmer for 1½ hours, removing scum that rises to top after first 15 minutes of cooking. Stir often to prevent sticking.

5. Turn off heat, cover, and let soup stand for one hour. Remove bouquet garni. Re-heat before serving.

YIELD: Serves 4; one portion left over

CAL	F	P:S	SOD	CAR	CHO
133.5	3	3.3:1	73.5	15	20

(18) Quick and Easy Sautéed Chicken Breasts

   1   tablespoon corn oil
   2   large shallots, minced
   2   large cloves garlic, minced
   ½   rib celery, finely minced
   1   teaspoon finely minced green pepper
   2   whole boneless chicken breasts, about 1½ pounds,
       each cut in half
   ½   teaspoon ground ginger
   8   dashes cayenne pepper
   ¼   cup dry vermouth
   ⅓   cup stock (page 187)
   1   tablespoon minced fresh tarragon, or 1½ teaspoons
       dried tarragon leaves, crushed
       Minced fresh parsley

1. Heat oil in large non-stick skillet until hot. Spread out shallots, garlic, and minced vegetables in skillet. Sauté for 1 minute.

2. Wash chicken and pat dry with paper toweling. Sprinkle with ginger and cayenne. Lay on sautéed mixture. Sauté over medium-high heat on both sides until lightly browned.

3. Add vermouth, and cook 1 minute.

4. Add stock and tarragon. Bring to simmering point. Cover and simmer gently for 15 minutes, turning and basting twice.

5. Remove from heat. Baste. Cover and let stand for 5 minutes before serving.

6. Serve on individually heated serving plates, spooning sauce over chicken. Sprinkle with parsley and serve.

YIELD: Serves 4

CAL	F	P:S	SOD	CAR	CHO
238.5	11	2:1	163	3.5	84

(19) Baked Sweet Rice

- 1 tablespoon corn oil, plus ¼ teaspoon to oil baking dish
- 1 small onion, minced
- 1 tablespoon finely minced green pepper
- 1 large clove garlic, minced
- ¾ cup rice
- 2 tablespoons dry vermouth
- 1 cup water, or cooking juices from your own vegetables
- ½ cup apple juice, no sugar added
- 6 whole cloves
- 1 teaspoon ground ginger
- ¼ teaspoon ground cinnamon
- 4 dashes cayenne pepper
- 2 teaspoons minced basil leaves, or 1 teaspoon dried basil leaves, crushed
- 1 small acorn squash, peeled, pulp and seeds removed, then diced
- 1 large, crisp, sweet apple, peeled, cored, and diced

1. Heat oil in non-stick skillet until hot. Sauté onion, pepper, and garlic until wilted but not brown.
2. Add rice, continuing to sauté for 1 minute.
3. Add vermouth, and cook 1 minute.
4. Add balance of ingredients, except apple. Bring to simmering point. Pour into 1¾-quart lightly oiled ovenproof casserole. Cover and bake in pre-heated 400° oven for 20 minutes.
5. Add apple, stirring into mixture. Re-cover and bake for 20 minutes.

YIELD: Serves 4; one portion left over

NOTE: Vegetable juices are more flavorful than water. Save cooking liquids from steamed or boiled vegetables.

CAL	F	P:S	SOD	CAR	CHO
248	3.6	4.5:1	22.5	47.5	0

(20) Sweet Baked Apples

    4 medium-sized baking apples, washed and cored
    ½ teaspoon grated lemon rind
    ¾ cup unsweetened pineapple juice
    1 tablespoon raisins
    1 teaspoon ground cinnamon
    ½ teaspoon ground ginger

1. Make several slits in skins of apples to depth of ⅓ of apple starting from top center. Arrange in small shallow baking dish.

2. Combine balance of ingredients in saucepan. Bring to simmering point and simmer for 5 minutes. Pour over apples in equal amounts. Cover loosely with aluminum foil.

3. Bake in pre-heated 350° oven for 40 minutes, basting 3 times. Remove from oven and let cool in baking dish.

4. Serve warm or chilled.

YIELD: Serves 4

CAL	F	P:S	SOD	CAR	CHO
109	0	—	8.5	26	0

(21) Curried Mushrooms on Toast

½ pound fresh mushrooms, washed, dried,
  trimmed, and sliced
⅔ cup stock (page 187) or water
2 tablespoons corn oil
2 cloves garlic, minced
2 shallots, minced
2 tablespoons unbleached flour
3 tablespoons dry vermouth
2 teaspoons curry powder, no salt or pepper added
3 dashes cayenne pepper
¼ teaspoon dried rosemary leaves, crushed
1 tablespoon minced fresh parsley
½–⅔ cup non-fat liquid milk
4 thin slices of 100% Whole Wheat Bread (page
  189) or Chewy Multi-Floured Bread (page 191)

1. Combine mushrooms and stock or water in small saucepan.
Bring to simmering point, partially cover, and simmer for 5 minutes.
Drain mushrooms, reserving liquid. Set mushrooms aside. Measure
out ⅔ cup liquid for this recipe. Store balance in freezer for future
use in sauces or soup.
2. Heat oil in heavy-bottomed saucepan until hot. Add garlic and
shallots, and sauté for 2 minutes.
3. Sprinkle with flour and cook for 1 minute, stirring constantly.
4. Whisk in vermouth, ⅔ cup cooking liquid, spices, and herbs.
Bring to simmering point. Gradually add milk, stirring constantly.
5. Add mushrooms and bring to simmering point.
6. Pour over just-toasted slices of bread, and serve.

YIELD: Serves 4

NOTES: *Other Uses for Curried Sauce:*
1. Pour over egg-white omlette (see *The Dieter's Gourmet Cookbook*).
2. Pour over steamed fish, and vegetables like cauliflower, asparagus, broccoli, potatoes, Brussels sprouts, green beans, and potatoes.
3. My breads are preferred, but you may use a commercial salt-free, low-calorie bread.

CAL	F	P:S	SOD	CAR	CHO
146	8	4.5:1	49.5	13.5	1.5
With Multi-Floured Bread:					
138	8	4.5:1	49	15.5	1.5

(22) Sautéed Steak with Wine

1½ pounds lean boned sirloin, 1″ thick
6 dashes cayenne pepper
½ teaspoon dried thyme leaves, crushed
1 tablespoon each corn oil and Italian olive oil,
  combined
2 large cloves garlic, finely minced
3 large shallots, finely minced
3 fresh mushrooms, washed, dried, trimmed,
  coarsely chopped
½ cup dry red wine
2 teaspoons minced fresh tarragon leaves

1. Wipe meat with paper toweling. Rub with cayenne and thyme.
2. Heat one tablespoon oil in iron skillet until hot. Add steak and sauté 7 minutes, or until lightly browned. Turn.
3. Add balance of oil, together with garlic, shallots, and mushrooms. Sauté 7 minutes, or until meat is brown on outside and pink inside. If mushroom mixture browns too rapidly, push to side of skillet, where heat is less intense. Transfer to carving board. Cover loosely with waxed paper.
4. Add wine to skillet, scraping bottom of skillet to loosen browned particles. Add tarragon. Cook over medium-high heat for 2-3 minutes, reducing liquid by ⅓.
5. While sauce is reducing, slice meat ⅜″ thick at an angle and arrange on individual warmed plates. Pour exuded juices from meat into skillet, stirring well. Spoon hot sauce over meat and serve immediately.

YIELD: Serves 4

VARIATION: In place of ½ cup wine, use ¼ cup each wine and stock (page 187).

NOTE: This dish tastes best with *fresh* herbs. If fresh tarragon isn't available, look for fresh basil or dill.

CAL	F	P:S	SOD	CAR	CHO
305	12	.9:1	119	6	20
Variation:					
303	12	.9:1	130.5	8	20

(23) Skillet-Browned Potatoes

4 medium-sized potatoes, peeled, each cut into 6
   pieces
1 tablespoon corn oil
2 large shallots, minced
2 large cloves garlic, minced
2 dashes cayenne pepper
½ teaspoon curry powder, no salt or pepper added
¼ teaspoon each dried marjoram and thyme leaves,
   crushed
1 tablespoon minced fresh parsley

1. Bring large saucepan of water to boil. Add potatoes, partially cover, and simmer for about 10 minutes. Potatoes should be slightly undercooked. Drain and let cool to room temperature.

2. Heat oil until hot in non-stick skillet. Add shallots and garlic, and sauté over medium-high heat for 1 minute.

3. Add potatoes, turning to coat. Sprinkle with cayenne, curry, and herbs.

4. Continue sautéeing and turning until browned on all sides. Your skillet will be virtually dry. Do not add additional oil. Serve immediately.

YIELD: Serves 4

CAL	F	P:S	SOD	CAR	CHO
120	3.5	4.5:1	12	19.5	0

(24) Poached Pears in Calvados with Spiced Meringue Topping

A very special treat!

For the pears:

4 d'Anjou pears, about 1¼ pounds, peeled, cut in half and cored

¼ cup apple juice, no sugar added

⅓ cup Calvados, plus 2 tablespoons per serving to pour over pears

3 whole cloves

2 dashes ground nutmeg

1 teaspoon flavorful honey (optional)

For the topping:

2 egg whites

Pinch of cream of tartar

2 tablespoons flavorful honey

2 dashes ground cloves

1 teaspoon finely grated orange rind

1. Select pears that are not quite ripe but not rock-hard. Place in wide saucepan (it's best if all pears are arranged in one layer), and add balance of ingredients. Bring to simmering point. Partially cover and simmer for 7-10 minutes or until fruit is firm, yet tender. Remove cover. Let cool in liquid. Discard cloves.

2. Beat egg whites with cream of tartar and ground cloves until almost stiff, using electric beater at high speed. While egg whites are beating, pour honey into small oven-proof dessert dish which has been set in saucepan of simmering water. Heat until warm and liquid.

3. Slowly dribble honey into almost stiffly beaten egg whites, continuing to beat at high speed until blended. Sprinkle with orange rind and continue beating until egg whites are stiff.

4. Serve individual pears in large dessert dish. Pour cooking liquid in equal amounts over each pear. Add Calvados. Spoon 2 heaping tablespoons of topping over each dish.

YIELD: Serves 4

NOTE: The topping alone is a fine accompaniment to applesauce, baked apple, and cakes.

CAL	F	P:S	SOD	CAR	CHO
140	0	—	8.5	34	0
With honey:					
155.5	0	—	9	38	0
Topping:					
39	0	—	28.5	8.5	0

(25) Spiced Griddle Cakes

¼ cup whole-wheat flour
½ cup unbleached flour
2½ teaspoons low-sodium baking powder (available in health-food stores)
½ teaspoon ground ginger
¼ cup toasted wheat germ, no sugar added
1 teaspoon corn oil
⅓ cup crushed pineapple in its own juice
1 teaspoon grated orange rind, preferably from navel orange
1 teaspoon vanilla extract
¾ cup buttermilk, no salt added
¼ teaspoon corn oil to brush on skillet
Cinnamon or honey (optional)

1. Sift flours, baking powder, and ginger into bowl. Add wheat germ and stir to blend.
2. Combine oil, pineapple, orange rind, and vanilla. Stir into flour mixture. Add buttermilk, a little at a time. Batter will be thick.
3. Heat large non-stick skillet until hot enough for a drop of water to bounce off. Brush lightly with oil for first batch of griddle cakes. Cook 3 or 4 griddle cakes at a time. Turn when edges brown and top bubbles. Cook until lightly browned and puffed up.
4. Serve sprinkled with cinnamon, or with your favorite honey.

YIELD: Serves 12 griddle cakes, 3″ in diameter

CAL	F	P:S	SOD	CAR	CHO
Per cake:					
62	4.5	4.5:1	6.5	12	.5
With cinnamon:					
No appreciable difference					
With honey:					
83	4.5	4.5:1	8.5	16	.5

(26) Sautéed Chinese-Style Ve

      2 tablespoons corn oil
     ½ pound fresh mushrooms, washed, dried, trimmed,
        and thickly sliced
      1 small green pepper, parboiled, dried, cut into slivers
      3 large cloves garlic, finely minced
      2 onions, thinly sliced
      1 cake bean curd (tofu), to weigh 8 ounces, drained,
        dried, and cut into 1" squares
      2 teaspoons each wine vinegar and apple-cider
        vinegar
     ¾ cup bean sprouts, drained and dried
     ½ cup stock (page 187)
     ½ teaspoon each turmeric, and crushed dried
        marjoram leaves
      1 teaspoon ground ginger
      4 dashes cayenne pepper
     ½ cup pineapple chunks in their own juice, drained
      1 teaspoon low-sodium soy sauce (optional; available
        in health-food stores)
      2 teaspoons arrowroot flour dissolved in 1 tablespoon
        water

1. Heat one tablespoon oil in non-stick skillet until hot. Add mushrooms and sauté for 2 minutes, stirring constantly. Transfer to dish and set aside.

2. Heat balance of oil in skillet. Add green pepper, garlic, and onions. Sauté 3 minutes, stirring constantly.

3. Add bean curd, and sauté until heated through.

4. Add vinegars and cook for 1 minute.

5. Add bean sprouts, stirring quickly.

6. Add stock, turmeric, marjoram, ginger, pepper, and sautéed mushrooms. Cook 1 minute over medium-high heat. Sprinkle with optional soy sauce.

7. Dribble in just enough dissolved arrowroot flour mixture to thicken sauce lightly. Stir well. Serve immediately.

YIELD: Serves 4

NOTE: Total cooking time after mushrooms have been sautéed is 5 minutes. That's to preserve the delicious crunchiness which is characteristic of gourmet Chinese cooking. So be sure you have all your ingredients set out before you begin.

CAL	F	P:S	SOD	CAR	CHO
144	8.5	4.5:1	23.5	15.5	0
With soy sauce:					
144	8.5	4.5:1	107	15.5	0

(27) Fluffy and Delicious Boiled Rice

1 cup water
1 cup stock (page 187)
1 cup rice, white or brown; see note
1 medium onion, minced
1 teaspoon apple-cider vinegar
1 tablespoon minced fresh dill, parsley, basil, or
  tarragon
6 dashes cayenne pepper

1. Bring water and stock to rolling boil in medium-sized saucepan. Add rice, onion, and vinegar. Bring to simmering point. Partially cover, and cook for 15-17 minutes if using enriched white rice, or 20-25 minutes if using short-grain brown rice. All water will be absorbed and rice will be moist and fluffy.

2. Toss with freshly minced herb of your choice and cayenne. Serve immediately.

YIELD: Serves 4

NOTE: I prefer the short-grain organic variety of brown rice (see page 219). For best results, soak washed rice first in the 2 cups of liquid. Then continue with recipe.

CAL	F	P:S	SOD	CAR	CHO
236	0	—	29.5	49.5	0

(28) Pasta with Curried Tomato Sauce

1½	tablespoons each corn oil and Italian olive oil, combined
3	medium onions, minced
5	large cloves garlic, minced
4	large shallots, minced
2	medium green peppers, minced
1	rib celery, minced
½	pound fresh mushrooms, washed, dried, trimmed, and thickly sliced
¾	cup dry vermouth
2½–3	pounds fresh tomatoes, cored, skinned, and cut into ½" chunks
3	tablespoons tomato paste, no salt added
3	tablespoons minced fresh basil leaves
1	teaspoon dried tarragon leaves, crushed
1	tablespoon curry powder, no salt or pepper added
6	dashes cayenne pepper
2	large bay leaves
¾	pound whole-wheat spaghetti, or enriched vermicelli made with durum wheat, no salt added
½	teaspoon per serving low-fat cheese, like Sap Sago, to sprinkle over pasta (optional) (page 248)

1. Heat oil in large iron skillet until very warm. Add next 5 ingredients, and sauté, stirring constantly, until lightly browned.

2. Add mushrooms and sauté for 2 minutes.

3. Add vermouth and cook for 1 minute.

4. Add balance of ingredients, except spaghetti and cheese, stirring well. Bring to simmering point. Partially cover and simmer for 1 hour, stirring from time to time. Uncover, and simmer for 15 minutes. This will reduce liquid and thicken sauce naturally.

5. Cook spaghetti in rapidly boiling water for 8 minutes. Drain well. Add to hot sauce, stirring to blend.

6. Serve in individual heated bowls. Serve cheese on side as an optional accompaniment.

YIELD: Serves 6

NOTES:

1. This sauce tastes best if prepared in an iron skillet. Stir constantly during Steps #1 and #2 so that additional oil is not needed to brown ingredients.

2. To serve 4, prepare ½ pound spaghetti and freeze ⅓ of sauce for another meal.

CAL	F	P:S	SOD	CAR	CHO
192	7	2.3:1	71	24	0

With Sap Sago:
No appreciable difference

(29) Tangy Buckwheat Brownies

¼ cup buckwheat flour
¾ cup plus 2 tablespoons unbleached flour
2 teaspoons low-sodium baking powder
1 tablespoon ground cinnamon
½ teaspoon ground ginger
1 tablespoon date powder (available in health-food stores)
2 tablespoons finely chopped walnuts
½ egg yolk
3 tablespoons corn oil, plus ½ teaspoon to oil baking pan
1 tablespoon flavorful honey
2 tablespoons finely grated orange rind
½ cup pineapple juice, no sugar added
¼ teaspoon almond extract
3 tablespoons low-fat plain yogurt
3 egg whites
½ teaspoon cream of tartar

1. Sift flours, baking powder, cinnamon, and ginger into bowl. Stir in date powder and walnuts. Set aside.

2. Combine egg yolk with oil, honey, orange rind, pineapple juice, and almond extract, whisking until blended. Stir in yogurt with wooden spoon. Add dry ingredients to this mixture, ¼ cup at a time, stirring with wooden spoon to blend.

3. Beat egg whites with cream of tartar until stiff. Fold into batter. Do not overfold.

4. Spoon and spread into lightly oiled 9″-square baking pan. Bake in pre-heated 375° oven until lightly browned and mixture comes away from the side of pan (25-30 minutes).

5. Remove from oven. Cool on rack for 10 minutes. Cut into 12 squares while still warm. Serve slightly warm or cooled.

YIELD: 12 brownies

CAL	F	P:S	SOD	CAR	CHO
102.5	3	3.7:1	10	12	11

Second Week's Recipes

(30) Jiffy Orange Muffins

- ¾ cup whole-wheat flour
- 2 tablespoons unbleached flour
- 3 teaspoons low-sodium baking powder (available in health-food stores)
- 2 tablespoons toasted wheat germ, no sugar added
- 2 tablespoons date powder (available in health-food stores)
- 1 cup uncooked old-fashioned rolled oats
- ½ teaspoon each ground ginger and cinnamon
- 1 egg white, ½ egg yolk, or 2 egg whites
- 3 tablespoons corn oil, plus 1 teaspoon to oil muffin pans
- ½ cup fresh orange juice
- ½ cup non-fat liquid milk
- 2 teaspoons grated orange rind, preferably from navel orange
- ½ cup raisins

1. Combine first 7 dry ingredients in large mixing bowl, stirring to blend.

2. In another bowl combine egg, oil, juice, milk, and orange rind, beating with fork to blend.

3. Pour liquid ingredients into dry ingredients, stirring with wooden spoon until all liquid is absorbed. Fold in raisins.

4. Half fill lightly oiled 3" muffin pans with batter. Bake in preheated 400° oven for 20-22 minutes. Muffins should be well browned.

5. Remove from oven, placing muffin pan on rack. Let cool for 5 minutes. Loosen around sides of each muffin with blunt knife and serve warm.

YIELD: 12 small muffins

VARIATION: ¼ cup coarsely chopped walnuts may be folded into batter before baking.

NOTE: If you prefer larger muffins, fill each cup almost to top for a yield of 9 large muffins.

CAL	F	P:S	SOD	CAR	CHO
135	3.5	3.4:1	9	15	1
With 2 egg whites:					
134	2.5	4.5:1	9.5	15	0
Variation:					
141	8.5	6.3:1	9.5	16.5	1
Variation with 2 egg whites:					
140	7.5	7.2:1	9.5	16.5	0

(31) One-Step Chilled Fruit Soup

    1   cup fresh ripe peaches, peeled and sliced
    ¼   cup non-fat liquid milk
    ¼   cup low-fat plain yogurt
    3   tablespoons dry-curd cottage cheese, no salt added,
        less than ½% milkfat
    2   slices navel orange, peeled and cubed
    2   dashes each ground cinnamon, ginger, and nutmeg

1. Combine ¾ cup peaches and balance of ingredients in blender. Purée for 1 minute. Add balance of peaches to each portion, and serve.

YIELD: Serves 2

VARIATIONS: Try the following fruit substitutions for peaches:

- Fresh berries in season
- One ripe banana
- Pineapple chunks in their own juice
- Fresh nectarines
- Fresh apricots

NOTE: This dish tastes best if prepared just before serving, and milk, fruit, and cheese are well chilled.

CAL	F	P:S	SOD	CAR	CHO
98.5	1	trace:1	82	10.5	3
With berries:					
86	1	trace:1	81	12	3
With bananas:					
96.5	1	trace:1	82	13	3
With pineapple:					
112	1	trace:1	79	22.5	3
With nectarines:					
107	1	trace:1	82	33	3
With apricots:					
159.5	1	trace:1	85	32.5	3

(32) Roast Orange Chicken

1	3-pound broiling chicken, skinned, wing tips removed
⅓	cup fresh orange juice
2	teaspoons grated orange rind, preferably from navel orange
1	tablespoon corn oil
¼	cup wine vinegar
1	large clove garlic, finely minced
2	large shallots, finely minced
1	tablespoon finely grated carrot
½	teaspoon dry mustard
1	teaspoon ground cinnamon
½	teaspoon each dried sage and rosemary leaves, crushed
2	dashes each ground cloves, nutmeg, and cinnamon
1	tablespoon minced fresh parsley

1. Wash and pat bird dry, inside and out, with paper toweling. Place in deep bowl.

2. Combine balance of ingredients in jar. Shake well. This is your marinade.

3. Pour marinade over chicken, spooning some into cavity. Turn to coat. Cover with aluminum foil and refrigerate at least 6 hours. Remove from refrigerator 1 hour before cooking.

4. Place chicken on rack in shallow roasting pan, reserving marinade. Cover loosely with aluminum foil. Roast in pre-heated 375° oven for 20 minutes. Uncover, and pour ½ of reserved marinade over bird. Cover and roast another 25 minutes. Pour balance of marinade over bird. Return to oven, covered, for 10 minutes. Baste. Roast uncovered for 5 minutes.

5. Cut into serving pieces and serve.

YIELD: Serves 4

NOTE: The technique I've devised in preparing skinned roast chicken produces a delicious moist bird. You will discover that it has far more flavor prepared *without* the skin than conventional roast chicken prepared *with* the skin.

CAL	F	P:S	SOD	CAR	CHO
261.5	11.5	2:1	85	4	143

(33) Stir-Fried Zucchini with Apples

    2 tablespoons corn oil
    2 large cloves garlic, minced
    2 large shallots, minced
    3 medium-sized zucchini, well scrubbed, sliced ⅜"
        thick
    2 green tart apples, peeled, cored, halved, and sliced
        ⅜" thick
   ½ teaspoon dried tarragon leaves, crushed
   ¼ teaspoon dried marjoram leaves, crushed
    2 dashes ground cinnamon
 4–5 dashes cayenne pepper
    1 teaspoon wine vinegar
    1 tablespoon minced fresh tarragon, basil, or parsley

1. Heat oil in large non-stick skillet until hot. Add garlic and shallots and sauté for one minute.

2. Add zucchini and apples. Sprinkle with dried herbs, cinnamon, and cayenne, and sauté, stirring often, until zucchini and apples begin to soften.

3. Add vinegar and continue sautéeing for 2 minutes. Total cooking time: about 8 minutes. Sprinkle with fresh tarragon and serve.

YIELD: Serves 4

CAL	F	P:S	SOD	CAR	CHO
113	7	4.5:1	15.5	9	0

(34) Sweet Stewed Prunes

1   12-ounce box pitted prunes, no preservatives added
1   slice orange, including peel
1   teaspoon ground cinnamon
¼   teaspoon ground allspice
4   whole cloves
½-¾ cup apple juice, enough to barely cover

1. Empty contents of can into small saucepan. Add balance of ingredients. Bring to simmering point. Cover and simmer for 5 minutes.

2. Turn off heat and let stand, covered, for 30 minutes. Prunes will absorb most of liquid. Discard orange. Transfer to glass container and refrigerate.

YIELD: 7-8 servings; allow 4-5 prunes per serving

CAL	F	P:S	SOD	CAR	CHO
7 servings:					
130.5	0	—	4	33.5	0
8 servings:					
114	0	—	3.5	29.5	0

(35) Striped Bass Steaks with Barbeque Sauce

2   striped bass steaks, cut from large fish, 1½ pounds,
     each cut in half along length of bone
2   tablespoons fresh lime juice
1   tablespoon corn oil, plus ½ teaspoon to oil baking
     dish
2   tablespoons finely minced green pepper
1   large clove garlic, finely minced
1   small onion, grated
½   carrot, peeled and grated
¼   cup each dry vermouth, and apple juice, no sugar
     added
1   tablespoon tomato paste, no salt added
1   teaspoon dry mustard
½   teaspoon each dried thyme leaves, crushed, and
     chili con carne seasoning, no salt or pepper added
4   dashes cayenne pepper
1   teaspoon flavorful honey (optional)

1. Wash fish and pat dry with paper toweling. Arrange in lightly oiled baking dish in one layer.

2. Combine balance of ingredients in small saucepan. Bring to simmering point and simmer for 10 minutes.

3. Spoon half of cooked sauce over fish. Broil 2″ from heat for 7 minutes. Turn carefully with spatula. Spread balance of sauce over fish, and broil for 6-7 minutes, or until fish flakes easily. Serve immediately.

YIELD: Serves 4

SERVING SUGGESTIONS FOR BARBEQUE SAUCE:

1. Using above recipe instructions, spread on any of the following fish: thick fillets or steaks of tile fish, codfish steaks, fillets or steaks of scrod, halibut steaks, thick fillets of lemon sole, thick fillets of flounder.

2. A delicious filling for egg-white omelette

3. Pour over boiled whole wheat pasta.

4. Pour over baked or boiled potatoes.

5. Serve in gravy boat to accompany broiled chicken, chops, or steaks.

6. Pour over sliced, reheated turkey or chicken.

CAL	F	P:S	SOD	CAR	CHO
Fish:					
180	4.4	.8:1	60	0	94.5
Barbeque sauce:					
81	7.5	4.5:1	32.5	10.5	0
With honey:					
86.5	7.5	4.5:1	33	13.5	0

(36) Watercress and Endive Salad

½ bunch crisp watercress, washed and patted dry
2 large endives (½ pound), washed and patted dry
3 sliced pimentos, drained, no salt added
Salad dressing of your choice (pages 184–186)

1. Arrange watercress and endives in decorative pattern on individual servings plates. Lay pimentos over arrangements.
2. Pour 2 tablespoons of any of my salad dressings over each portion on salad just before serving.

YIELD: Serves 4

CAL	F	P:S	SOD	CAR	CHO
14	0	—	8	2.5	0
Zesty Salad Dressing:					
220	22	3:1	3	1	0
Curried Cottage Cheese Dressing:					
188	0	—	42	2	0
Tomato Salad Dressing:					
70	7	4.5:1	2	3	0

(37) Puffed Wheat Cookies

3 tablespoons corn oil, plus ¼ teaspoon to oil baking sheet
1 egg white, ½ egg yolk
2 tablespoons flavorful honey
1 teaspoon grated orange rind
1½ teaspoons vanilla extract
½ teaspoon almond extract
¼ cup buttermilk, no salt added
½ cup whole-wheat flour
⅓ cup unbleached flour
2 tablespoons date powder (available in health-food stores)
⅓ cup toasted wheat germ, no sugar added
2 teaspoons low-sodium baking powder
1 teaspoon ground cinnamon
1⅓ cup puffed wheat, no salt or sugar added

1. Combine oil, egg, honey, orange rind, and extracts in mixing bowl. Blend well with fork. Stir in buttermilk.
2. Combine flours, date powder, wheat germ, baking powder, and cinnamon in small bowl. Stir to blend. Add, a little at a time, to moist ingredients, stirring with wooden spoon after each addition.
3. Fold in puffed wheat.
4. Drop by spoonfuls onto lightly oiled baking sheet, pressing flat with moistened spoon. Bake in pre-heated 375° oven for 12 minutes. Transfer to rack and let cool. Let cookies stand, uncovered, for several hours before storing in tightly covered tin.

YIELD: 30 cookies

NOTE: Cookies may be crisped up next day, if necessary, by baking for 7 minutes in pre-heated 400° oven.

CAL	F	P:S	SOD	CAR	CHO
40	2	3.9:1	4	5	4

(38) Boston Salad

1 small head Boston lettuce, leaves separated, well
  washed, patted dry
½ bunch crisp watercress, well washed, leaves only,
  patted dry
1 endive, thinly sliced crosswise
2 scallions, minced
½ carrot, peeled and grated

1. Arrange lettuce leaves in circular pattern on individual salad plates. Place equal amounts of watercress in center of dish, and surround with endive slices.

2. Sprinkle center with scallions and carrot. Serve with your choice of salad dressing (pages 184–186), allowing 2 tablespoons per portion.

YIELD: Serves 4

VARIATIONS: For luncheon, add one of the following to each portion:

- 2 hard-boiled egg whites
- 1 portion fresh fruit, sliced
- heaping tablespoon dry-curd cottage cheese, no salt added, less than ½% milkfat
- 2 ounces cooked sliced chicken or meat
- 2 small cooked red-skinned potatoes, peeled and sliced

CAL	F	P:S	SOD	CAR	CHO
23.5	0	—	17	5	0
With egg whites:					
31.5	0	—	44.5	5	0
With fruit:					
45.5	0	—	17.5	9	0
With cottage cheese:					
27.5	0	—	32	5.5	.5
With chicken:					
43	1	1:2	27.5	0	11
With meat:					
45	1	trace:1	32	0	17
With potatoes:					
44.5	0	—	19	8	0

(39) Frothy Fruit Milk Shake

½ small banana
¼ cup apple juice, no sugar added
3 tablespoons low-fat plain yogurt
⅓ cup non-fat liquid milk
¼ teaspoon vanilla extract, or few drops almond extract
3 dashes each ground ginger and cinnamon
3 crushed ice cubes

1. Combine all ingredients in blender, and blend on high speed for one minute.

YIELD: One tall glass milk shake

VARIATIONS: Replace banana with one of the following:

- 1 small fresh peach or nectarine, peeled and sliced
- ¼ cup berries in season, washed and patted dry
- ¼ cup pineapple chunks in their own juice

CAL	F	P:S	SOD	CAR	CHO
172	0	—	39	30.5	2.5
With peach:					
108.5	0	—	35	18	2.5
With nectarine:					
114.5	0	—	26	22	2.5
With berries:					
96.5	0	—	48	18	2.5
With pineapple:					
109.5	0	—	33	22.5	2.5

(40) Broiled Curried Veal Chops

    4 loin or rib veal chops, about 1½ pounds, well
       trimmed
    3 large shallots, finely minced
    2 cloves garlic, minced
    1 teaspoon dried rosemary leaves, crushed
    4 dashes cayenne pepper
    1 tablespoon combined corn oil and Italian olive oil
 1½ tablespoons wine vinegar
    1 tablespoon minced fresh parsley
    2 teaspoons curry powder, no salt or pepper added
    1 tablespoon stock (page 187), optional
       Minced fresh parsley

1. Pat chops dry with paper toweling. Combine balance of ingredients, except parsley, blending well.
2. Spread ½ of mixture over chops. Place on rack in shallow broiling pan and broil 2″ from heat, coated side up, for 8-10 minutes.
Turn, spread with balance of mixture, and broil 8-10 minutes, or
until lightly browned. Meat should remain pink inside. Broiling time
will vary with thickness of chops. Sprinkle with parsley and serve.

YIELD: Serves 4

HEALTH HINT: Do not cook well-done. Overcooking destroys nutri-
tive value by 50%.

CAL	F	P:S	SOD	CAR	CHO
309	15.5	1.5:1	140.5	5	153
With stock					
314.5	15.5	1.5:1	149	5.5	160

(41) Quick-Cooking Kasha (Buckwheat Groats)

½   cup stock (page 187)
¼   cup apple juice, no sugar added
1–1¼ cups water
1   cup kasha (use the variety designated "whole")
2   cloves garlic, minced
1   teaspoon apple-cider vinegar
2   large shallots, minced
2   tablespoons minced fresh dill or basil
1   tablespoon grated carrot
4   dashes cayenne pepper
¼   teaspoon smoked yeast (available in health-food stores; optional)

1. Bring stock, apple juice, and one cup water to rolling boil in medium-sized saucepan. Add kasha, garlic, and vinegar. Cook, uncovered, over medium-high heat (liquid should continue to slow-boil—not simmer) for exactly 8 minutes. All liquid will be absorbed. Add balance of water, if necessary, to complete prescribed cooking time.

2. Toss gently with balance of ingredients. Serve immediately.

YIELD: Serves 4

NOTE: This dish tastes best prepared just before serving in order to retain its nut-like flavor and textured consistency.

CAL	F	P:S	SOD	CAR	CHO
114	0	—	32	25.5	0

(42) Sweet French Toast

    4   slices salt-free bread, sliced ½" thick
    3   egg whites
    ½   egg yolk
    ¼   cup apple juice, no sugar added
    ¼   cup non-fat liquid milk
    4   dashes ground cinnamon
    2   dashes each ground allspice and cayenne pepper
    3   teaspoons corn oil
        Cinnamon or honey (optional)

1. Soak bread in combined mixture of eggs, apple juice, milk, and spices which have been beaten with fork to blend. Let stand until most of liquid is absorbed.

2. Heat 2 teaspoons oil in large non-stick skillet until hot. Add bread slices, pouring any unabsorbed liquid over them. Sauté over medium-high heat until brown on both sides, adding balance of oil just before turning.

3. Serve immediately, sprinkled with cinnamon or spooned with honey.

YIELD: Serves 4

NOTE: Try Chewy Multi-Floured Bread (page 191) for a stick-to-the-ribs French Toast.

CAL	F	P:S	SOD	CAR	CHO
With Multi-Floured Bread:					
99.5	8	3.1:1	38	7	32

(43) Chilled Baby Bean Salad

1 cup small white beans (baby beans)
3 tablespoons Zesty Salad Dressing (page 184)
¼ teaspoon chili con carne seasoning, no salt or
   pepper added
1 tablespoon fresh lemon juice
2 tablespoons minced fresh parsley
4 dashes cayenne pepper
1 large pimento, no salt added, cut into strips

1. Soak beans overnight in water to cover. Drain. Add to pot of boiling water and cook, partially covered, until tender. Drain. Transfer to bowl and let cool.

2. Combine salad dressing, chili con carne seasoning, lemon juice, parsley, and cayenne in jar, shaking well. Pour over cooled beans, tossing gently.

3. Add pimentos, stirring to blend. Serve well chilled.

YIELD: Serves 4

SERVING SUGGESTION: Excellent as a luncheon dish served on a bed of lettuce, or to be included in cold buffet

CAL	F	P:S	SOD	CAR	CHO
192.5	4	3:1	26	28	0

(44) Simple Lemon Curry Chicken

1½ pounds boneless chicken breasts, skinned, cut into
    serving pieces
⅓ cup fresh lemon juice
3 tablespoons unsweetened pineapple juice
2 tablespoons dry vermouth
½ teaspoon each ground ginger and turmeric
4 dashes cayenne pepper
1 teaspoon curry powder, no salt or pepper added
2 teaspoons coriander seeds, finely crushed
2 cloves garlic, minced
1 medium onion, minced
1 tablespoon grated carrot
3 tablespoons raisins
1 tablespoon flavorful honey (optional)

1. Pat chicken dry with paper toweling.

2. Combine and stir balance of ingredients (except honey) in heavy aluminum kettle or waterless cooker. Add chicken, turning well to coat. Cover. Let stand for 30 minutes.

3. Bring to a simmer, and cook for 40 minutes, turning 3 times. Turn off heat. Let stand for 30 minutes.

4. Re-heat just before serving, adding honey if desired.

YIELD: Serves 4

CAL	F	P:S	SOD	CAR	CHO
264	8.5	1:1	112	17	101
With honey:					
279.5	8.5	1:2	112.5	19	101

(45) Apple Whip

  2 cups very cold applesauce (page 100)
  2 tablespoons Calvados or Apple Jack
  2 egg whites
  ¼ teaspoon ground cinnamon
  3 dashes each ground cloves and allspice
  1 dash nutmeg

1. Prepare applesauce ahead of time so that it is well chilled. In a bowl, combine applesauce with liqueur, blending well.
2. Beat egg whites until stiff, sprinkling in spices toward the end of beating process.
3. Whisk ½ of egg-white mixture into applesauce. Fold in balance. Spoon into 6 chilled dessert dishes and serve.

YIELD: Serves 6

CAL	F	P:S	SOD	CAR	CHO
48.5	0	—	23	10	0

(46) Prune Whip

    1 recipe Stewed Sweet Prunes (page 134)
    ¼ cup chopped California dates
    ¼ cup apple juice, no sugar added (optional)

1. Prepare prunes according to directions, adding dates to saucepan.
2. Purée in food mill. Stir to blend. If thinner consistency is desired, add small amount of apple juice, blending well. The apple juice will also increase the sweetness of the whip.

YIELD: About 1¼ cups; serves 5-6.

CAL	F	P:S	SOD	CAR	CHO
Serves 5:					
209	0	—	6.5	53	0
Serves 6:					
174	0	—	5.5	44	0

(47) Apple Pancakes

1 egg white, ½ egg yolk
1 tablespoon corn oil, plus ½ teaspoon to brush on skillet
½ cup apple juice, no sugar added
½ cup buttermilk, no salt added
1 teaspoon vanilla extract
1 teaspoon grated lemon rind
¾ cup whole-wheat flour
½ cup unbleached flour
3 teaspoons low-sodium baking powder
½ teaspoon ground cinnamon
¼ teaspoon each ground ginger and allspice
1 dash ground cloves
¼ cup toasted wheat germ, no sugar added
  Cinnamon or honey (optional)

1. Break egg. Drop white into small bowl of mixing machine, and ½ of yolk into another bowl. Discard balance of yolk.
2. Add 1 tablespoon oil to yolk and blend with whisk. Add apple juice, buttermilk, vanilla, and lemon rind, blending well.
3. Sift flours, baking powder, and spices into yolk mixture, a little at a time, stirring after each addition. Stir in wheat germ.
4. Beat egg white until stiff. Gently fold into mixture.
5. Allowing ½ cup batter per pancake, pour and spread into lightly oiled, well-heated, non-stick omelette skillet and cook until browned. Turn and cook until lightly browned. Serve immediately, sprinkled with cinnamon or spread with flavorful honey.

YIELD: 4 large pancakes: serves 4

NOTE: A ¼ cup low-fat plain yogurt and ¼ cup non-fat liquid milk, combined, may be substituted for buttermilk.

CAL	F	P:S	SOD	CAR	CHO
274	7	2.9:1	35.5	38	32
With cinnamon:					
No appreciable difference					
With honey:					
289.5	7	2.9:1	40	42.5	32
With yogurt and non-fat milk:					
283.5	8.5	2.9:1	50.5	47	34

(48) Gray Sole Paupiettes

1½   pounds thin fillets of gray sole, or baby sole
1½   tablespoons fresh lime juice
½   teaspoon ground ginger
1   teaspoon fresh basil, minced, or ½ teaspoon dried
    basil leaves, crushed
1   tablespoon finely grated low-fat cheese, like Sap
    Sago (page 248)
4   dashes cayenne pepper
2   cloves garlic, finely minced
2   large shallots, finely minced
2   tablespoons minced fresh parsley
½   cup apple juice, no sugar added
3   tablespoons dry vermouth
½   teaspoon corn oil
½   teaspoon grated orange rind, preferably from navel
    orange
2   teaspoons arrowroot flour dissolved in 1
    tablespoon water

1. Wash fillets and pat dry with paper toweling. Rub on both sides with lime juice. Sprinkle with ginger and basil, pressing into fillets. Sprinkle on one side with cheese. Roll up and secure with toothpicks. Sprinkle with cayenne.

2. Pre-heat oven to 450° for 10 minutes. Place paupiettes in lightly oiled casserole in one layer.

3. Combine garlic, shallots, 1 tablespoon parsley, apple juice, and vermouth in saucepan. Bring to simmering point. Pour over fish. Heat casserole on top of stove until liquid starts to simmer, spooning liquid over fish.

4. Turn oven heat down to 400°. Place casserole, uncovered in oven and bake for 6 minutes. Turn fish carefully and baste. Return to oven and bake 7-8 minutes more, or until fish flakes easily. Do not overcook. Transfer paupiettes to covered serving dish.

5. Add orange rind to liquid in casserole. Bring to simmering point and gently simmer for 2 minutes. Pour exuded juices from fish into sauce. Whisk in arrowroot flour mixture, using only enough to thicken lightly.

6. Pour sauce over paupiettes. Sprinkle with balance of minced parsley and serve.

YIELD: Serves 4

NOTE: Cooking time may vary slightly depending upon thickness of fillets.

CAL	F	P:S	SOD	CAR	CHO
175	8	2.5:1	142.5	8	94.5

Baby sole:
No appreciable difference.

(49) Gingered Rice and Carrots

  1   tablespoon corn oil
  3   large shallots, minced
1½   cups cooked brown rice
  4   medium carrots, peeled, cubed, and cooked
  ½   teaspoon ground ginger
  3   dashes cayenne pepper
  1   teaspoon rosemary leaves, crushed
  ¼   cup apple juice, no sugar added
  1   tablespoon minced fresh parsley

1. Heat oil in non-stick skillet until hot. Add shallots and sauté for one minute.
2. Add rice and carrots. Sprinkle with ginger, cayenne, and rosemary. Stir until well heated.
3. Add apple juice, a tablespoon at a time, stirring well.
4. Serve piping hot, sprinkled with parsley.

YIELD: Serves 4

NOTE: This dish tastes best if rice and carrots are prepared *al dente* (firm-textured) and ingredients are assembled just before serving.

CAL	F	P:S	SOD	CAR	CHO
223	3.5	4.5:1	53.5	40.5	0

(50) Broiled Tomatoes

2 large ripe tomatoes, cored
1 teaspoon each corn oil and Italian olive oil,
  combined
2 teaspoons grated onion
4 dashes cayenne pepper
2 teaspoons minced fresh tarragon or basil
3 teaspoons crumbs, made with 2 teaspoons toasted
  bread crumbs and 1 teaspoon toasted wheat germ,
  no sugar added

1. Lay tomatoes on their sides and cut in half, placing knife between top and bottom. Arrange, skin side down, in lightly oiled baking dish.
2. Brush with half of oil; spoon on grated onion. Then sprinkle with cayenne, fresh tarragon or basil, and bread crumbs. Dribble balance of oil over tops of tomatoes.
3. Place under pre-heated broiler, 2″ from heat, and broil until tender (about 10 minutes).

YIELD: Serves 4

CAL	F	P:S	SOD	CAR	CHO
40.5	2.5	2.8:1	4.5	4	0

(51) Skillet Meatballs with Savory Sauce

1 pound lean beef, like shoulder steak or top round, ground
2 tablespoons toasted wheat germ, no sugar added
¼ cup chopped sweet peeled apple
4 dashes cayenne pepper
1 tablespoon minced fresh basil
½ teaspoon grated orange rind, preferably from navel orange
1 tablespoon corn oil
2 large cloves garlic, finely minced
1 small onion, finely minced
1 tablespoon finely minced green pepper
2 tablespoons dry vermouth
2 tablespoons fresh lemon juice
⅓ cup each stock (page 187) and apple juice, no sugar added
1 tablespoon each honey and wine vinegar
½ teaspoon ground ginger
  Minced fresh basil or parsley

1. Combine meat with wheat germ, apple, 2 dashes cayenne pepper, basil, and orange rind in small bowl.
2. Heat ½ of oil in non-stick skillet until hot. Sauté garlic, onion, and green pepper until lightly browned. Add vermouth and cook for 1 minute.
3. Pour into meat mixture, blending well. Shape into 16 balls. Wipe out skillet.
4. Heat balance of oil in skillet until hot. Sauté meatballs until lightly browned on all sides, pouring off any accumulated fat.
5. Combine lemon juice, stock, apple juice, honey, and vinegar. Pour over browned meatballs. Sprinkle with balance of cayenne and ginger. Bring to simmering point. Cover and simmer gently for 30 minutes, turning twice.
6. Turn into serving dish. Sprinkle with basil or parsley and serve.

YIELD: Serves 4

SERVING SUGGESTION: Delicious served over Quick-Cooking Kasha (page 142)

NOTE: Fresh herbs taste best in this dish. If fresh basil isn't available, substitute fresh dill for 5th ingredient.

CAL	F	P:S	SOD	CAR	CHO
313	12	1.3:1	130	11	120

(52) Minted Peas

1½	pounds fresh peas, shelled
1	tablespoon corn oil
1	clove garlic, minced
1	shallot, minced
4	large fresh mushrooms, washed, dried, trimmed, and thickly sliced
3–4	dashes cayenne pepper
1	teaspoon minced fresh mint leaves
¼	teaspoon marjoram leaves, crushed
	Minced fresh parsley

1. Boil peas in water to cover for 8 minutes. Drain. Color should remain bright green.

2. Heat oil in non-stick skillet until hot. Add garlic, shallot, and mushrooms, and sauté until lightly browned.

3. Add peas. Sprinkle with cayenne and herbs and shake in circular motion.

4. Serve immediately, sprinkled with minced fresh parsley.

YIELD: Serves 4

CAL	F	P:S	SOD	CAR	CHO
179.5	3.5	4.5:1	8	26.5	0

(53) Apple Whip Sherbet

1   recipe Apple Whip (page 146)

1. Prepare apple whip. Turn into freezer tray and freeze (do not allow tray to rest on metal in freezer compartment).
2. Whisk in tray every hour 3 times. Freeze another hour and serve.

YIELD: Serves 6

CAL	F	P:S	SOD	CAR	CHO
48.5	0	—	23	10	0

(54) Creamy Egg Salad

    4 hard-boiled eggs
    2 tablespoons finely minced onion
    1 small rib celery, finely minced
    1 teaspoon minced fresh tarragon
    5 dashes cayenne pepper
    2 teaspoons Zesty Salad Dressing (page 184)
    ¼ teaspoon ground ginger
    2 teaspoons low-fat plain yogurt

1. Cut eggs in half. Discard all yolks but ½ of one egg yolk. Mash egg yolk and egg white together with fork.
2. Add balance of ingredients except yogurt, stirring to blend.
3. Stir in yogurt. Serve well chilled.

YIELD: Serves 4

SERVING SUGGESTIONS:
1. As a salad, serve on lettuce leaves, surrounded with fresh fruit or crisp fresh vegetables.
2. Serve as an open-faced sandwich spread on 4 slices of any of my breads, thinly sliced, garnished with slivers of green pepper and pimentos.
3. Serve as a canapé spread on 4 slices of any of my breads, cutting each slice into quarters. Garnish with pimentos.

NOTE: My breads are preferred, but you may use a low-salt, low-calorie commercial bread.

CAL	F	P:S	SOD	CAR	CHO
62.5	8.5	1.7:1	41	2	42.5
Per sandwich:					
98	7	1.9:1	33.5	12	32
Per canapé:					
24.5	2	1.9:1	8.5	3	8
As a salad:					
See Diet for Life Foods, page 205.					

(55) Caraway Cheese Dip

  6 tablespoons dry-curd cottage cheese, no salt added,
     less than ½% milkfat
  1 tablespoon low-fat plain yogurt
  ½ teaspoon caraway seeds, well crushed
  2 teaspoons minced fresh parsley
  4 dashes cayenne pepper
  2 tablespoons crushed pineapple in its own juice, well
     drained

In small bowl, mash cheese together with yogurt, caraway seeds, parsley, and cayenne. Stir in pineapple. Chill. Spread on toasted unsalted rice or wheat wafers.

YIELD: ¾ cup; allow one teaspoon per dip

VARIATION: This is a tasty filling for hard-boiled egg whites, celery, or crisp endive leaves.

CAL	F	P:S	SOD	CAR	CHO
1.5	0	—	7	.5	0

Variation:
See Diet for Life Foods, page 205.

(56) Mushroom and Rice Patties

½ cup brown rice
½ cup stock (page 187)
1 cup water
1 ½"-thick slice salt-free bread, lightly toasted and cubed
¼ cup non-fat liquid milk
1 tablespoon corn oil
2 large fresh mushrooms, washed, dried, trimmed, and coarsely chopped
2 large cloves garlic, minced
2 large shallots, minced
1 tablespoon finely grated carrot
1 tablespoon minced fresh dill
1 small egg white lightly beaten with fork
2 teaspoons tomato paste, no salt added
¼ teaspoon ground ginger
⅛ teaspoon paprika
3 dashes cayenne pepper
¼ teaspoon dried thyme leaves, crushed

1. Bring stock and water to rolling boil. Add rice, partially cover, and simmer slowly until all liquid is absorbed. Turn into bowl. Let cool.

2. Place bread in small dish. Pour milk over it and mash. Let stand a few minutes until all milk is absorbed.

3. Heat ½ of oil in non-stick skillet until hot. Add mushrooms, garlic, and shallots. Sauté for 3 minutes, adding carrot during last minute of cooking.

4. Pour sautéed ingredients into rice, together with softened bread and balance of ingredients, blending well with spoon. Cover and refrigerate until well chilled. Mixture may be prepared ahead of time up to this point and refrigerated several hours before sautéing.

5. Shape into 8 small patties. Heat balance of oil in skillet until hot. Sauté patties until browned on both sides. Serve immediately.

YIELD: 8 patties; serves 4

NOTES:

1. My breads are preferred, but you may use a commercial low-salt, low-calorie bread.

2. Cooking juices (1½ cups) from your own vegetables make an excellent substitute for stock.

CAL	F	P:S	SOD	CAR	CHO
Using my Multi-Floured Bread:					
298.5	3.5	4.5:1	45	52	.5

(57) Pineapple-Banana Mousse

¾ cup pineapple juice, liquid from 20-ounce can
   pineapple chunks in their own juice
¼ cup apple juice, no sugar added
⅓ cup combination raisins and unsweetened chopped
   dates
1 tablespoon plain gelatin or 1 pre-measured package
1 20-ounce can pineapple chunks in their own juice,
   drained
⅛ teaspoon each ground cinnamon and ginger
1 teaspoon fresh lemon juice
¼ teaspoon almond extract
1 small banana (about 4 ounces)
4 tablespoons low-fat plain yogurt
2 egg whites, stiffly beaten with pinch of cream of
   tartar

1. Combine pineapple and apple juice together with raisins and dates in small saucepan. Bring to boil. Turn heat down, and simmer for 5 minutes. Add gelatin, stirring to dissolve. Cool.

2. Place pineapple chunks, spices, lemon juice, and almond extract in blender. Add cooled gelatin mixture and blend for 1 minute. Pour into bowl.

3. Mash banana with fork. Add yogurt and blend. Whisk into puréed mixture. Refrigerate until well chilled and mixture begins to thicken.

4. Whisk ⅓ of stiffly beaten egg whites into thickened mixture. Fold in balance.

5. Spoon into 6 dessert dishes and chill until set (about 3 hours).

YIELD: Serves 6

VARIATION: Sprinkle each serving with ½ teaspoon coarsely chopped walnuts.

CAL	F	P:S	SOD	CAR	CHO
73	.5	trace:1	28.5	3	0
With walnuts:					
86	2	9:1	28.5	3.5	0

162

(58) Steamed Artichokes with Vinaigrette Dressing

For the Vinaigrette Dressing:
- 1   tablespoon each corn oil and Italian olive oil
- ¼   cup each wine vinegar and apple-cider vinegar
- 2   tablespoons tomato juice, no salt added
- 1   tablespoon grated onion
- 1   large shallot, finely minced
- ½   teaspoon paprika
- 4   dashes cayenne pepper
- 2   teaspoons minced fresh parsley
- 1   teaspoon minced fresh tarragon or basil

For the artichokes:
- 4   medium-sized artichokes, well washed and trimmed of tough outer leaves, stem removed
- ¼   teaspoon dried thyme leaves, crushed
- 2   tablespoons fresh lemon juice
- 1   clove garlic, finely minced
- 1   shallot, finely minced

1. Prepare dressing first. Combine all ingredients in jar, shaking to blend. Let stand until artichokes are cooked. Shake again before serving.

2. Arrange artichokes in saucepan, stem-side down. Add 2″ of water and balance of ingredients. Bring to simmering point. Cover and simmer until tender (about 45 minutes), spooning with liquid from time to time. Drain.

3. Serve, either hot or chilled, with dressing on the side.

YIELD: Serves 4; about ¾ cup dressing. Allow 2 tablespoons per serving.

CAL	F	P:S	SOD	CAR	CHO
Artichoke:					
54.5	0	—	43.5	40.5	0
Dressing:					
60	6	2.9:1	6	1	0

(59) Succulent Broiled Flounder

4 whole fresh baby flounders, about ¾ pound each, cleaned
¼ cup wine vinegar
½ teaspoon each dried rosemary and thyme leaves, crushed
1 tablespoon corn oil
3 large cloves garlic, finely minced
3 large shallots, finely minced
1 small rib celery, finely minced
2 tablespoons minced fresh parsley
6 dashes cayenne pepper
   Several sprigs crisp watercress
   Lemon wedges

1. Wash fish and pat dry inside and out with paper toweling. Make 3-4 diagonal gashes across each fish on each side.

2. Combine next 8 ingredients in jar, shaking to blend. This is your marinade.

3. Lay fish in shallow broiling pan. Pour marinade over fish, turning to coat, spooning some into cavities. Cover and refrigerate for 2 hours before broiling.

4. Remove fish from marinade. Drain. Lay on rack in broiling pan. Strain marinade, discarding liquid. Strew half of minced ingredients retained in strainer over fish, pressing into gashes.

5. Broil under medium-high heat for 8 minutes. Turn. Strew balance of minced ingredients over fish. Broil for 7-8 minutes, or until fish flakes easily when tested with fork. Do not overcook.

6. Serve each fish on individual plates garnished with watercress and lemon wedges.

YIELD: Serves 4

CAL	F	P:S	SOD	CAR	CHO
309.5	6	2.5:1	88	2	22

(60) One-Bowl Mystery Cake

    1   whole egg, or ½ egg yolk and 2 egg whites
    1   tablespoon flavorful honey
    2   tablespoons corn oil, plus ½ teaspoon to oil pan
    1   teaspoon vanilla extract
    ½   teaspoon almond extract
    ½   cup low-fat plain yogurt
    ¼   cup apple juice, no sugar added
    ¾   cup chopped Stewed Sweet Prunes, drained (page
        134)
    ¼   cup toasted wheat germ, no sugar added
    ½   cup whole-wheat flour
    ¾   cup unbleached flour
    2   teaspoons low-sodium baking powder
    ¼   teaspoon allspice
    1½ teaspoons ground cinnamon
    ½   teaspoon ground ginger
    2   tablespoons coarsely chopped walnuts

1. Whisk together egg, honey, and oil in bowl. Stir in extracts.
2. Combine yogurt and apple juice and add to mixture. Stir in prunes and wheat germ.
3. Sift flours, together with baking powder and spices, into moist ingredients. Stir with wooden spoon until all flour is absorbed.
4. Pour into lightly oiled loaf pan (7⅜″ x 3⅝″ x 2¼″). Sprinkle with nuts. Bake in pre-heated 350° oven for 1 hour. Cake is done when toothpick inserted into center comes out dry.
5. Place pan on rack to cool for 10 minutes. Using blunt knife, loosen around sides and invert. Let cool completely before slicing.

YIELD: 10 slices

CAL	F	P:S	SOD	CAR	CHO
160.5	5.5	3:1	21.5	23	28
With ½ egg yolk and 2 egg whites:					
159.5	4.5	3:1	26.5	23	15

(61) Fruit Chiffon Mold

½   cup buttermilk, no salt added
½   cup pineapple juice, no sugar added
1   tablespoon fresh lime juice
½   teaspoon ground ginger
¼   teaspoon anise seed, well crushed
1   cup dry-curd cottage cheese, no salt added, less
    than ½% milkfat
2   envelopes unflavored gelatin
½   cup apple juice, no sugar added
¾   cup drained pineapple tidbits in their own juice, or
    pineapple chunks, each chunk cut in ½
1   egg white, stiffly beaten
    Several crisp lettuce leaves to line serving plate
1½ cups combined diced fresh fruit and berries
2   tablespoons coarsely chopped walnuts (optional)

1. Combine buttermilk, juices, ginger, seeds, and cottage cheese in blender. Purée for 20 seconds. Pour into bowl.

2. Soften gelatin in apple juice. Warm and stir until gelatin is dissolved. Cool.

3. Pour gelatin mixture into blended mixture, whisking to blend. Chill until slightly thickened.

4. Fold in pineapple. Then gently fold in egg white.

5. Rinse a 1-quart ring or decorative mold with cold water. Fill with mixture. Chill until firm.

6. Unmold by dipping mold into warm water for 30 seconds. Invert onto lettuce-lined plate. If using ring mold, fill center with mixed fruit. If using decorative mold, arrange fruit around mold. Sprinkle with nuts.

YIELD: 4 luncheon servings; 8 salad servings

CAL	F	P:S	SOD	CAR	CHO
Luncheon serving:					
119.5	0	–	111	13	3.5
With walnuts:					
132.5	1.5	9:1	118.5	13.5	3.5
Salad serving:					
60	0	–	55.5	6.5	2
With walnuts:					
69.5	1	9:1	60.5	6.5	0

(62) Chicken with Yams

    2 boneless chicken breasts, skinned, each cut in ½
    2 legs with thighs, skinned, legs separated from thighs
    1 recipe marinade from Roast Orange Chicken (page
       132)
    2 teaspoons corn oil
    1 medium onion, sliced
    ¼ cup apple juice, no sugar added
    2 medium yams, peeled, cut into ½" slices
    4 dashes cayenne pepper

1. Pat chicken dry with paper toweling. Prepare marinade in bowl large enough to accommodate all chicken pieces. Add chicken, turning to coat. Cover, refrigerate, and marinate for at least 4 hours.

2. Drain chicken, reserving marinade. Pat dry with paper toweling. Heat oil in iron skillet until hot. Add chicken and onion. Sauté both together until browned.

3. Add marinade, apple juice, yams, and cayenne. Bring to simmering point. Add chicken, turning to coat. Cover and bake in preheated 375° oven for 45 minutes, turning twice.

4. Remove from oven and let stand for 20 minutes. Re-heat briefly on top of stove before serving.

YIELD: Serves 4

CAL	F	P:S	SOD	CAR	CHO
319	12	2.7:1	93.5	18.5	56.5

(63) Tart Savoy Cabbage

  1 head savoy cabbage, about 1 pound
  ¼ cup apple juice, no sugar added
  ⅓ cup grape juice, no sugar added
  4 whole cloves
  ¼ teaspoon ground allspice
  4 dashes cayenne pepper
  ½ teaspoon chili con carne seasoning, no salt or
     pepper added
  1 teaspoon fresh lemon juice
  1 tablespoon apple-cider vinegar

1. Cut cabbage into quarters, cutting away hard center section. Arrange in small waterless cooker or heavy kettle.
2. Combine balance of ingredients and pour over cabbage. Bring to boil. Turn heat down to simmering point. Cover tightly and simmer for 45 minutes, spooning liquid over cabbage several times.
3. Turn off heat and let stand for 20 minutes. Re-heat and serve.

YIELD: Serves 4

CAL	F	P:S	SOD	CAR	CHO
47.5	0	—	25	10.5	0

(64) Crunchy Chicken Salad

                3   cups cooked chicken, cut into ½" cubes
                1   tablespoon fresh lime juice
                1   medium carrot, peeled and grated
                1   rib celery, diced
                1   small onion, thinly sliced
                1   small crisp apple, peeled, cored, and diced
              4–6   tablespoons salad dressing (pages 184–186)
                ⅛   teaspoon ground ginger
                4   dashes cayenne pepper
                1   tablespoon minced fresh tarragon, basil, or dill
                ½   pound fresh peas, cooked and cooled
                1   tablespoon coarsely chopped walnuts or almonds
                    (optional)

1. Place chicken in large bowl together with lime juice. Toss well.
2. Add carrot, celery, onion, and apple. Pour only enough salad dressing over mixture to moisten. Stir to blend. Sprinkle with ginger and cayenne.
3. Gently fold in tarragon, peas, and nuts.

YIELD: Serves 4 as main course; enough for 8 sandwiches

NOTE: Eggless low-sodium mayonnaise may be substituted for salad dressing.

CAL	F	P:S	SOD	CAR	CHO
With Zesty Salad Dressing:					
281	17.5	2.5:1	102.5	28	54
With Tomato Salad Dressing:					
206	10	2.4:1	102	14.5	54
With eggless mayonnaise:					
242	8	2.8:1	105	14	0
With almonds, add:					
120	11	2.5:1	3	4	0
With walnuts, add:					
144	14	9:1	60	4	0

(65) Marinated Beef with Vegetables

For the meat and marinade:

- 1 pound lean tender beef, like flank steak, well trimmed
- ¼ cup dry vermouth
- ¼ cup unsweetened apple juice
- 1 tablespoon fresh lemon juice
- 1 teaspoon ground ginger
- 1 teaspoon chili con carne seasoning, no salt or pepper added

For the vegetables and sauce:

- 1½ tablespoons corn oil
- 3 large cloves garlic, minced
- 1 small green pepper, cut into ⅛" slivers
- 2 large onions, thinly sliced
- 3 large scallions, cut diagonally into ½" chunks
- ¼ pound fresh mushrooms, washed, dried, trimmed, and thickly sliced
- 6 dashes cayenne pepper
- ½ teaspoon smoked yeast (available in health-food stores) (optional)
- ¾ teaspoon chili con carne seasoning, no salt or pepper added
- ½ teaspoon each dried rosemary and thyme leaves, crushed
- ½ cup stock (page 187)
- 1½ tablespoons tomato paste, no salt added

1. Wipe meat with paper toweling. Cut into ½" strips.
2. Combine balance of ingredients, for marinade, in bowl. Add meat, turning to coat. Cover and let stand for 30 minutes.
3. Heat ½ of oil in non-stick skillet until hot. Add garlic, green pepper, onions, and scallions. Sauté over high heat for 3 minutes, stirring constantly. Push vegetables to side of skillet. Add mushrooms and sauté for 2 minutes. Combine all ingredients in skillet.
4. Sprinkle with cayenne, smoked yeast, chili con carne seasoning, and dried herbs.
5. Combine stock and tomato paste. Add to mixture, stirring to blend. Bring to simmering point and simmer for 30 seconds. Pour into covered casserole dish. Wipe out skillet.
6. Heat balance of oil in skillet until hot. Add meat. Sauté over

high heat for 30 seconds or less on each side. Lay meat on top of hot vegetables and sauce, and serve.

YIELD: Serves 4

NOTE: Steps 3 through 6 are done in rapid succession. Have all ingredients measured and ready for each step before you start to cook.

CAL	F	P:S	SOD	CAR	CHO
Meat and marinade:					
175	5.5	trace:1	123	2	102
Vegetables and sauce:					
70	5	4.5:1	40	10	0

(66) Mocha Sponge

1½ cups non-fat liquid milk
1 envelope unflavored gelatin
1 tablespoon decaffeinated coffee, or coffee
   substitute
1 tablespoon carob powder, no sugar added
½ teaspoon ground cinnamon
4 dashes ground nutmeg
1 tablespoon flavorful honey
½ cup apple juice, no sugar added
1 teaspoon vanilla extract
2 egg whites, stiffly beaten with pinch of cream of
   tartar

1. Pour milk into small saucepan. Add gelatin. Stir. Heat slowly, together with coffee, carob, spices, and honey until ingredients are dissolved. Do not boil. Add apple juice, stirring to blend.

2. Pour into bowl and cool. Stir in vanilla. Refrigerate until mixture begins to thicken.

3. Fold in egg whites.

4. Spoon into 6 dessert dishes and chill until set.

YIELD: Serves 6

CAL	F	P:S	SOD	CAR	CHO
52	0	–	80.5	6	1.5

(67) Curried Tomato-Pea Soup

1½ tablespoons combined corn oil and Italian olive oil
1½ cups minced onions
 3 large cloves garlic, minced
 1 large rib celery, minced
 1 tablespoon apple-cider vinegar
2½ pounds fresh ripe tomatoes, cored and chopped
 ¾ cup split peas, washed
 1 cup each stock (page 187) and water
 ½ cup tomato purée, no salt added
 2 tablespoons minced fresh basil or parsley
 ½ teaspoon dried rosemary leaves, crushed
 ¼ teaspoon dried thyme leaves, crushed
 1 bay leaf
 2 tablespoons curry powder, no salt or pepper added
 1 tablespoon minced fresh parsley for garnish

1. Heat oil in stainless-steel pot or waterless cooker. Add onions, garlic, and celery and sauté over medium heat until wilted.

2. Add vinegar and cook 1 minute.

3. Add balance of ingredients, except parsley. Bring to boil. Turn off heat. Cover. Let stand for 1 hour.

4. Re-heat to simmering point, partially cover, and cook for 1 hour. Let soup cool in pot. Discard bay leaf.

5. Pour into blender and purée for 1 minute. Re-heat and serve, sprinkled with parsley.

YIELD: Serves 6

VARIATION: Whisk in ⅓ cup low-fat plain yogurt to blended cooled mixture. Serve chilled.

CAL	F	P:S	SOD	CAR	CHO
182	20	2.9:1	25	24	0
Variation:					
185.5	20	2.9:1	32	25	1

(68) Crisp and Moist Fillets of Lemon Sole

1½ pounds fresh fillets of lemon sole
2 teaspoons minced fresh dill or parsley
⅓ cup dry vermouth
1 tablespoon each wine vinegar and fresh lime juice
6 dashes cayenne pepper
1 large clove garlic, minced
2 large shallots, minced
⅓ cup matzoh crumbs
2 tablespoons corn oil
Lemon wedges

1. Wash fish and pat dry with paper toweling. Cut into serving pieces.
2. Combine next 6 ingredients in shallow dish. Add fillets, turning to coat. Marinate for 1 hour at room temperature, turning often.
3. Drain fillets. Dip into crumbs, coating well on both sides.
4. Using 2 large non-stick skillets, heat 1 tablespoon oil in each skillet until hot. Add ½ of fillets to each skillet and sauté on both sides to a golden brown. Total cooking time is about 12 minutes.
5. Garnish with lemon wedges and serve.

YIELD: Serves 4

NOTE: Fillets of gray sole or flounder may be substituted for lemon sole.

CAL	F	P:S	SOD	CAR	CHO
162.5	8	4:1	136	3.5	99.5
Gray sole or flounder: No appreciable difference					

(69) Stuffed Cornish Hens with Grape Sauce

For the hens and basting sauce:
- 2 Cornish hens, fresh, if possible, 1½ pounds each
- 2 teaspoons fresh lime juice
- 2 teaspoons corn oil to brush on hens and oil roasting pan
- ¼ teaspoon each dried rosemary and sage leaves, crushed
- ¼ teaspoon ground ginger
- 4 dashes cayenne pepper
- 2 large shallots, minced
- ¼ cup stock (page 187)
- ⅓ cup grape juice, no sugar added
- 1 teaspoon fresh lemon juice
- 2 tablespoons dry vermouth
- 1 tablespoon minced fresh parsley

For the stuffing:
- ¼ cup raw brown rice
- 2 teaspoons corn oil
- 1 tablespoon minced onion
- 1 large clove garlic, minced
- 1 large shallot, minced
- 1 tablespoon finely minced celery
- 2 fresh mushrooms, washed, dried, trimmed, and coarsely chopped
- ¼ teaspoon each dried rosemary and thyme leaves, crushed
- ¼ teaspoon ground ginger
- 5 dashes cayenne pepper
- ½ sweet crisp apple, peeled and coarsely chopped
- 1 tablespoon minced fresh parsley

1. Skin hens, trimming away fat. Wash inside and out under cold running water. Pat dry with paper toweling. Rub cavity and outside of hens with lime juice. Cover and refrigerate until ready to stuff.

2. Prepare stuffing next. Cook rice in boiling water, partially covered, for 15 minutes. Rice will be undercooked. Drain.

3. Heat oil in non-stick skillet until hot. Sauté onion, garlic, shallot, celery, and mushrooms until wilted. Sprinkle with herbs and spices. In small bowl, combine cooked rice with sautéed ingredients, apple, and parsley.

4. Pat hens lightly with paper toweling. Stuff cavities with rice mixture and secure with poultry skewers. Tie ends of legs together

with thread. Brush lightly with oil. Then sprinkle with crushed herbs and spices. Lightly oil shallow roasting pan and sprinkle with minced shallot. Lay hens, breasts down, on shallot. Roast in pre-heated 450° oven for 10 minutes.

5. Prepare basting sauce by combining stock, grape juice, lemon juice, vermouth, and parsley in small saucepan. Heat.

6. Reduce oven heat to 375°. Turn hens on their backs. Spoon with ¼ of basting sauce. Cover with aluminum foil and roast for 20 minutes. Spoon with ¼ basting sauce every 20 minutes 3 times more, each time re-covering with aluminum foil. Total cooking time is 1½ hours.

7. Transfer hens to cutting board. Remove poultry skewers and thread. Cut each hen in half. Lay, stuffing side down, on individual warmed plates. Turn heat up under roasting pan on top of stove and cook sauce for 2 minutes, stirring constantly. Spoon over birds and serve.

YIELD: Serves 4

NOTE: This dish makes an extravagant festive main course. I suggest that you study the entire recipe carefully before starting preparation.

CAL	F	P:S	SOD	CAR	CHO
Hens and basting sauce:					
242.5	10	1.8:1	64.4	2.2	107.5
Stuffing:					
100	2.5	4.5:1	15	16	0

(70) Grape Sherbet

1¼ cups apple juice, no sugar added
2 teaspoons grated orange rind, preferably from
   navel orange
1½ teaspoons unflavored gelatin
1 cup grape juice, no sugar added
2 egg whites, stiffly beaten

1. Heat ½ cup apple juice in saucepan together with orange rind. Bring to boil, then simmer for 2 minutes. Add gelatin, stirring to dissolve. Pour into large bowl. Cool.

2. Add balance of apple juice to mixture together with grape juice. Stir to blend.

3. Pour into freezer tray, placing tray directly on metal base of freezer compartment. Freeze until thick and mushy. Transfer to chilled bowl and whisk until mixture is smooth and fluffy.

4. Add egg whites as follows: whisk ⅓ of egg whites into mixture. Fold in balance. Return to freezer tray and freeze. Remove from freezer after 1 hour. At this point top has started to solidify and bottom is liquid. Fold bottom over top with spoon until most of liquid is absorbed.

5. Repeat freezing and folding process every hour twice more. Whisk in freezer tray until smooth. Return to freezer. Sherbet will be fully ripened in flavor and ready to serve 5-6 hours from starting point.

YIELD: Serves 6

CAL	F	P:S	SOD	CAR	CHO
64.5	0	–	14	18	0

(71) Chili Pork Chops

    4 loin or rib pork chops, ½″ thick, well trimmed, 1½
      pounds
    1 tablespoon corn oil
    ⅓ cup combination wine vinegar and apple-cider
      vinegar
    2 large cloves garlic, finely minced
    ¼ cup fresh orange juice
    2 tablespoons fresh lime juice
    1 tablespoon grated onion
    1 tablespoon finely minced green pepper
    1 tablespoon finely grated carrot
    ¼ teaspoon each ground ginger and crushed thyme
      leaves
    2 teaspoons chili con carne seasoning, no salt or
      pepper added

1. One hour before cooking time, wipe chops with paper toweling. Place in bowl.
2. Combine balance of ingredients in jar, shaking well. This will be your broiling sauce.
3. Pour sauce over chops, spreading evenly to coat. Mixture will be thick. Cover and let stand for 1 hour.
4. Pre-heat broiler. Place chops on rack in broiling pan, reserving sauce. Broil 1½″ from heat for 5 minutes. Turn. Spoon with sauce and broil for 5 minutes. Continue broiling, turning, and spooning with sauce until chops are done (about 20 minutes). Do not overcook. Serve immediately.

YIELD: Serves 4

NOTE: This chili broiling sauce doubles as a marinade for roast or broiled chicken. Follow cooking directions on pages 105 and 132.

CAL	F	P:S	SOD	CAR	CHO
358	19.5	3.3:1	121	3	154

(72) Sweet Potato-Apple Mélange

2 large sweet potatoes, about one pound, well
   scrubbed, cut in half
2 crisp sweet apples, peeled and cut into ⅜″ slices
2 teaspoons corn oil
2 large shallots, minced
½ teaspoon each ground cinnamon and ginger
5 dashes cayenne pepper
⅓ cup combined fresh orange juice and pineapple
   juice, no sugar added, warmed
2 whole cloves
1 tablespoon minced fresh parsley

1. Parboil potatoes in water to cover for 7 minutes. Let cool. Peel
and cut into ⅜″ slices.
2. Arrange potatoes and apples in 2-quart oven-proof casserole in
alternate layers, sprinkling oil, shallots, and spices between layers.
Pour fruit juices over mixture. Add cloves and sprinkle with parsley.
3. Cover and bake in pre-heated 400° oven for 20-25 minutes, or
until tender, stirring once midway.

YIELD: Serves 4

CAL	F	P:S	SOD	CAR	CHO
131	2.5	4.5:1	17.5	44	0

(73) Baked Stuffed Eggplant

1 eggplant, about 1 pound
1 tablespoon combined corn oil and Italian olive oil
2 large cloves garlic, minced
3 large shallots, minced
1 small onion, minced
3 large fresh mushrooms, washed, dried, trimmed, and coarsely chopped
2 tablespoons finely minced green pepper
2 ripe fresh tomatoes, skinned, cored, and cubed
2 tablespoons tomato paste, no salt added
2 tablespoons dry vermouth
4 dashes cayenne pepper
½ teaspoon each ground ginger and dried marjoram leaves, crushed
2 tablespoons minced fresh basil

1. Wash and dry eggplant. Cut in half lengthwise. Insert serrated knife ¼″ from skin. Cut around entire vegetable in a scooping motion and remove pulp, taking care not to break shell. Cut pulp into ½″ cubes.

2. Heat oil in non-stick skillet until hot. Sauté eggplant, garlic, shallots, onion, mushrooms, and green pepper over medium-high heat until lightly browned.

3. Add tomatoes and tomato paste, stirring to blend. Add vermouth. Bring to simmering point. Stir in spices, marjoram, and one tablespoon basil.

4. Pile into shells. Place in baking dish that has been filled with ½″ hot water. Bake in pre-heated 375° oven for 20-25 minutes, or until eggplant shell is tender. Cut each piece in half. Sprinkle with balance of basil and serve.

YIELD: Serves 4 as side dish; serves 2 as main dish

VARIATION: Sprinkle with 2 teaspoons low-fat Sap Sago cheese just before serving.

NOTE: Minced fresh parsley and dill may be substituted for basil.

CAL	F	P:S	SOD	CAR	CHO
108	3.5	2.8:1	16.5	17.5	0

Variation:
No appreciable difference

(74) Buttermilk Coleslaw

4 cups thinly sliced tender green cabbage
2 tablespoons finely minced green pepper
1 tablespoon finely minced onion
1 tablespoon grated carrot
2 tablespoons wine vinegar
1 tablespoon apple-cider vinegar
2 tablespoons apple juice, no sugar added
4–6 dashes cayenne pepper
¼ teaspoon ground ginger
2 tablespoons minced fresh dill and parsley
¾ cup thick buttermilk, no salt added

1. Combine first 4 ingredients in large bowl.
2. Add vinegars and apple juice and toss.
3. Sprinkle with spices and herbs, tossing again.
4. Add buttermilk, a little at a time, stirring and turning after each addition. Cover with plastic wrap and refrigerate for several hours before serving, stirring often.

YIELD: Serves 6

CAL	F	P:S	SOD	CAR	CHO
35	0	—	13.5	2	1

(75) Fallen Angel Food Cake with Berry Topping

For the cake:

- ¼ cup date powder (available in health-food stores)
- ¼ cup carob powder, no sugar added (available in health-food stores)
- ½ cup unbleached flour
- 8 egg whites
- 1 teaspoon cream of tartar
- 1 teaspoon vanilla extract
- 2 teaspoons orange rind, preferably from navel orange

For the berry topping:

- 1¼ cups fresh sweet berries in season
- ½ teaspoon grated lemon rind
- ¼ cup low-fat plain yogurt
- ¼ teaspoon almond extract
- ½ teaspoon vanilla extract
- ½ teaspoon ground cinnamon
- 1 tablespoon flavorful honey (optional)

1. Pour date powder into blender and blend until pulverized to the consistency of powder. Combine with flour and carob powder. Sift 4 times, discarding particles of date powder that don't sift through.

2. Beat egg whites and cream of tartar with large wire whisk or with electric beater with whisk attachment. It's necessary to incorporate as much air as possible during the beating process. Add orange rind, ¼ teaspoon at a time, while still beating. Add vanilla. Continue beating until stiff.

3. Fold 2 tablespoons of dry mixture at a time into beaten egg whites. Do not overfold. Turn into ungreased 9" tube pan.

4. Bake in pre-heated 350° oven for 40 minutes, or until delicately browned. Invert pan and let cool completely on rack. Loosen sides and around tube with spatula. Lift the tube section out of pan. Then loosen bottom of pan with spatula and lay cake on rack to cool.

5. To prepare topping, mash berries with fork in small bowl. Add balance of ingredients, blending well. Place in freezer compartment of refrigerator for 1 hour. Spoon over cake.

YIELD: Serves 8

CAL	F	P:S	SOD	CAR	CHO
Cake:					
102.5	0	–	56.5	19	0
Topping:					
17.5	.5	trace:1	10.5	4	4
With honey:					
25	.5	trace:1	10.5	5	4

*Basic Recipes for Steaming Vegetables,
Making a Trio of Salad Dressings, Cooking
Stock, and Baking Three Kinds of Breads*

Steamed Vegetables
(Basic Recipe)

1. Arrange one or more vegetables, cut uniformly, in steamer. Steam until just tender. Do not overcook.

2. Season with 2 teaspoons fresh lemon juice, cayenne pepper to taste, and 2 tablespoons freshly minced herbs of your choice.

NOTES:

1. When cooking broccoli, promote tenderness and reduce bitterness by peeling off the skin from the stalk and flowerettes.

2. The following vegetables steam well together:

- Carrots and potatoes
- Green beans and carrots
- Cabbage and potatoes
- Sweet potatoes and white potatoes
- Turnip and carrots

Zesty Salad Dressing

⅓ cup combined apple-cider vinegar and wine vinegar
⅓ cup each corn and Italian olive oil
2 shallots, finely minced
½ teaspoon dried mustard
6 dashes cayenne pepper
½ teaspoon dried thyme leaves, crushed
2 teaspoons minced fresh basil or tarragon

1. Combine all ingredients in jar, and shake well. Let stand for 1 hour before using. Shake again before serving.

YIELD: 1 cup

NOTES:
1. Fresh herbs contribute to a superior salad dressing. If fresh basil and tarragon are unavailable, substitute minced fresh dill.
2. This dressing will keep well, refrigerated, for 4 days. Remove from refrigerator 1 hour before serving.

CAL	F	P:S	SOD	CAR	CHO
Per tablespoon:					
110	11	3:1	1.5	.5	0

Curried Cottage Cheese Dressing

⅓ cup dry-curd cottage cheese, no salt added, less than
   ½% milkfat
2 tablespoons low-fat plain yogurt
½ cup tomato juice, no salt added
1 tablespoon finely minced onion or scallion
2 teaspoons fresh lemon juice
1 teaspoon curry powder, no salt or pepper added
1 teaspoon minced fresh tarragon or dill
4 dashes cayenne pepper

1. Combine all ingredients in blender, and purée for 30 seconds. Chill. This is excellent served on cold vegetables, salads, and with cold fish.

YIELD: 1 cup

NOTE: This dressing will keep well, refrigerated, for 3 days.

CAL	F	P:S	SOD	CAR	CHO
Per tablespoon:					
10	0	—	21	1	0

Tomato Salad Dressing

⅔ cup tomato juice, no salt added
¼ cup corn oil
2 tablespoons fresh lemon juice
½ teaspoon ground ginger
2 shallots, finely minced
4 dashes cayenne pepper
1 teaspoon each minced fresh tarragon and parsley

1. Combine all ingredients in jar, and shake well. Let stand for one hour before using. Shake again before serving.

YIELD: 1 cup

NOTES:
1. Fresh herbs contribute to a superior salad dressing. If fresh tarragon is not available, substitute minced fresh dill.
2. This dressing will keep well, refrigerated, for 4 days. Remove from refrigerator 1 hour before serving.

CAL	F	P:S	SOD	CAR	CHO
Per tablespoon:					
35	3.5	4.5:1	1	1.5	0

All-Purpose Stock

2	pounds chicken giblets, backs and wings, or chicken parts, skinned
2	pounds veal knuckles, cracked
1	large carrot, peeled and cut into 4 pieces
4	large cloves garlic, coarsely chopped
2	large shallots, coarsely chopped
2	onions, quartered
1	leek, white part only, washed, trimmed, and coarsely chopped
1	small white turnip, peeled and diced
4	large fresh mushrooms, washed, trimmed, and thickly sliced
2	ribs celery, each cut into 4 pieces
2–2½	quarts water, just enough to cover
½	cup dry vermouth
4	dashes cayenne pepper
	Large bouquet garni

1. Remove all skin from chicken and casings from necks. Trim off fat and discard. Wash well. Rinse cracked bones well.

2. Place bones and chicken parts in large kettle or waterless cooker no wider than 9″ in diameter. Add water to cover. Bring to vigorous boil, and continue boiling for 2 minutes. Pour contents of kettle into colander and rinse scum from chicken and bones.

3. Return bones and chicken to pot. Add balance of ingredients. Bring to simmering point, partially cover, and continue simmering for 2½-3 hours, removing scum periodically. Turn off heat, and let cool in pot.

4. Pour into a chinois (a utensil for draining and pressing out juices), placing bowl underneath, and press on ingredients with back of wooden spoon to remove all stock. Transfer stock to freeze-proof containers. Cover loosely with waxed paper, and cool at room temperature.

5. Cover tightly, and refrigerate overnight. Then cut away and discard hardened fat from top of stock. Refrigerate some of stock for use within 3-4 days, covering tightly, and freeze the balance.

YIELD: About 2 quarts

NOTE: This stock works beautifully in all recipes in this book calling for stock.

CAL	F	P:S	SOD	CAR	CHO
Per cup:					
66	0	—	98	3.5	0

100% Whole-Wheat Bread

2 tablespoons dry yeast, or 2 pre-measured
  packages
2 tablespoons toasted wheat germ, no sugar added
1 tablespoon anise seeds, crushed
6–6½ cups whole-wheat flour
1 teaspoon each ground ginger and cinnamon
1¼ cups water
1 cup apple juice, no sugar added
1 tablespoon corn oil, plus 1 teaspoon to oil
  utensils
2 teaspoons grated orange rind
1 tablespoon honey (optional)
⅔ cup low-fat plain yogurt, room temperature

1. In large bowl of mixing machine, combine and stir yeast, wheat germ, seeds, 2 cups flour, and spices.

2. Heat water, apple juice, oil, orange rind, and optional honey until warm (105°-115°). Pour over dry ingredients and mix with wooden spoon. Beat with electric beater on medium speed for 1 minute, or with wooden spoon for 2 minutes.

3. Add yogurt and beat again until blended.

4. Add 4 cups of flour, ½ cup at a time, beating well with wooden spoon after each addition. When mixture becomes too difficult to handle with spoon, turn onto lightly floured board. Knead until smooth and elastic. Add balance of flour if dough is still sticky and knead until smooth.

5. Shape into a ball. Drop into lightly oiled, fairly straight-sided bowl. Turn to coat. Cover with plastic wrap and let rise at room temperature (70°-80°) until double in bulk (about 1½ hours). Hint for faster rising: fill your rising bowl with hot water, pour out water, dry well before coating with oil.

6. Punch dough down and knead briefly. Shape into ball. Cut in half. Press out all bubbles, and shape into loaves. Place in two small lightly oiled loaf pans (7⅜" x 3⅝" x 2¼"). Cover loosely with waxed paper and let rise until double in bulk.

7. Bake in pre-heated 375° oven for 45 minutes. Remove loaves from pans. Place on rack in oven, and bake another 5 minutes. Remove from oven. Bread is completely baked when you tap bottom with knuckles and hear a hollow sound. Place on rack and cool thoroughly before slicing.

YIELD: 3 loaves; twenty ⅜" slices per loaf

CAL	F	P:S	SOD	CAR	CHO
Per slice:					
51	.5	3.9:1	2.5	10	0
With honey:					
52	.5	3.9:1	3	10.5	0

Chewy Multi-Floured Bread

2	tablespoons dry yeast, or 2 pre-measured packages
1½	cups medium rye flour
1	cup whole-wheat flour
3½	cups unbleached flour
¾	cup gluten flour
2	tablespoons toasted coriander seeds, crushed
1	teaspoon anise seeds, crushed
½	cup pineapple juice, no sugar added
1	tablespoon corn oil, plus 1 teaspoon to oil utensils
1½	cups water
1	teaspoon grated orange rind, preferably from navel orange
1	cup buttermilk, no salt added, room temperature
3	tablespoons toasted wheat germ, no sugar added
1	tablespoon white cornmeal
1	egg white mixed with 1 teaspoon water

1. In large mixing bowl, combine and stir yeast, ½ cup rye flour, ½ cup whole-wheat flour, one cup unbleached flour, all of gluten flour, and seeds.

2. Heat pineapple juice, oil, water, and orange rind until warm (105°-115°). Pour into dry mixture and beat on medium speed of mixing machine for 2 minutes.

3. Add buttermilk and continue beating for 2 minutes.

4. Add balance of whole-wheat and rye flours, 2 cups unbleached flour, and wheat germ, ½ cup at a time, beating well after each addition with wooden spoon.

5. When dough can no longer be handled with spoon, scoop up and turn onto lightly floured board and knead, using balance of flour, if necessary, until dough is smooth, elastic, and no longer sticky. This may take a bit of doing because of the volume of dark flours, but stay with it and the stickiness will disappear. This thorough kneading process is vital for a digestible, well-risen loaf.

6. Lightly oil a large, fairly straight-sided bowl. Shape dough into smooth ball and drop into bowl, turning to coat. Cover with plastic wrap, and let rise at room temperature (70°-80°) until double in bulk (about 1¼ hours).

7. Punch dough down, kneading out bubbles. Cut in half. Shape into 2 high, smooth loaves. Very lightly rub baking sheet (11½" x 15½") with oil, then sprinkle with cornmeal. Place loaves in opposite corners. Brush with egg-white mixture. Cover loosely with waxed paper and let rise until double in bulk (about 1 hour).

8. Brush again with egg-white mixture. Bake in pre-heated 375°

oven for 45 minutes. Tap bottom of loaves with knuckles. They're fully baked when you hear a hollow sound. Let cool on rack thoroughly before slicing.

YIELD: 2 loaves. Each ¼ loaf makes eight ½" uneven slices.

CAL	F	P:S	SOD	CAR	CHO
Per slice:					
39	.5	3.9:1	2	18	0

Raisin Bread

> 2 tablespoons dry yeast, or 2 pre-measured packages
> ½ cup warm water (105°-115°)
> 1 cup apple juice, no sugar added
> ¾ cup water
> 2 tablespoons corn oil, plus 1 teaspoon for oiling utensils
> 1 tablespoon grated orange rind, preferably from navel orange
> 1½ cups whole-wheat flour
> 3½ cups unbleached flour
> ½ cup wheat germ, no sugar added
> ⅓ cup non-fat dry milk
> 1 teaspoon anise seeds, lightly crushed
> ½ teaspoon each ground ginger and cinnamon
> ¾ cup raisins

1. Combine yeast and ½ cup warm water in large bowl of mixing machine. Beat with fork to blend. Let stand for 10 minutes.

2. Heat apple juice, ¾ cup water, oil, and orange rind until warm (105°-115°). Stir into yeast mixture.

3. Combine flours, wheat germ, non-fat dry milk, anise, and spices. Add 3 cups of flour mixture to liquid, beating with wooden spoon until blended. Cover and let stand for 15 minutes.

4. Add raisins and stir to blend.

5. Add all but ½ cup flour mixture, ½ cup at a time, beating well with wooden spoon after each addition. When dough can no longer be handled with spoon, scoop up and turn onto lightly floured board and knead, using balance of flour, if necessary, until smooth and elastic.

6. Shape into ball. Drop into lightly oiled, fairly straight-sided bowl. Turn to coat. Cover with plastic wrap and let rise at room temperature (70°-80°) until double in bulk. Punch dough down, and shape into ball. Cut into thirds. Shape into 3 loaves. Place in lightly oiled small loaf pans (7⅜" x 3⅝" x 2¼"). Cover loosely with waxed paper and let rise until double in bulk.

7. Bake in pre-heated 375° oven for 45 minutes. Remove from pans. If bottoms of loaves are not well browned, place back on oven rack and bake for 5 minutes more. Remove from oven and let cool thoroughly on rack before slicing.

YIELD: 3 loaves; 15 slices

NOTE: Because there is no sugar or honey added to these loaves, they taste best the first or second day. I recommend cutting surplus loaves into ⅜" slices, reassembling into loaf shape, wrapping tightly in aluminum foil, and freezing. Then whenever you want a fresh-tasting slice of toast, just flip off a slice, pop it into your toaster, and—*voilà!*

CAL	F	P:S	SOD	CAR	CHO
Per slice:					
62	.5	4.5:1	3.5	10.5	0

For Condiment Lovers

All-Round Sauce

½   cup tomato purée, no salt added
¼   cup tomato juice, no salt added
1   teaspoon each corn oil and Italian olive oil
1   tablespoon each fresh lime and lemon juice
1   tablespoon wine vinegar
1   tablespoon grated onion
1   large shallot, finely minced
2   teaspoons chili con carne seasoning, no salt or
    pepper added
¼   teaspoon dry mustard
2   teaspoons minced fresh parsley
½   teaspoon low-sodium soy sauce (available in health-
    food stores) (optional)
4   dashes cayenne pepper

1. Combine and stir all ingredients in jar. Let stand 1 hour before using to develop flavor.
2. Store, refrigerated, in glass jar. Stir before using.

YIELD: About 1 cup. Allow 2 tablespoons per serving.

NOTE: May be refrigerated and kept up to 4 days

CAL	F	P:S	SOD	CAR	CHO
Per tablespoon:					
20	1.5	2.9:1	5	3	0
With low-sodium soy sauce:					
27	1.5	2.9:1	9	3	0

My Ketchup

½ cup tomato purée, no salt added
1 tablespoon tomato paste, no salt added
4 dashes each cayenne pepper and nutmeg
¼ teaspoon ground ginger
2 teaspoons freshly minced parsley
1 teaspoon honey

1. Combine all ingredients, stirring to blend. Store in glass jar in refrigerator.

YIELD: ⅔ cup. Allow 2 tablespoons per serving.

NOTE: May be refrigerated and kept for up to 4 days.

CAL	F	P:S	SOD	CAR	CHO
Per tablespoon:					
10	0	—	2.5	2.5	0

8

How to Convert Your Favorite Recipes to Diet for Life Recipes

It's a simple two-step process.

Step 1. Replace the forbidden (potentially harmful) ingredients in your favorite recipe—or in any new recipe you want to try—with favored (healthful) ingredients. When there's no replacement for a forbidden ingredient, simply eliminate it.

Step 2. To heighten taste appeal, add flavorsome herbs, spices, juices, vinegars, and wine.

To carry out *Step 1 for cooking,* make use of the list of *Forbidden* and *Favored* ingredients, which starts on this page. *For baking,* make use of the lists starting on page 202 (for cakes and cookies) and on page 204 (for bread).

To carry out *Step 2 for cooking,* model your conversions on the sample converted recipes for a beef dish (page 200), a fish dish (page 202), and a poultry dish (page 201). *For baking,* follow the guidelines beginning on page 202. For both cooking and baking, read through my recipes in this book to get the feel of my techniques. Do write me, in care of the publisher (the address is on the reverse side of the title page), and tell me how your conversions worked out.

Forbidden and Favored Ingredients for Cooking

FORBIDDEN INGREDIENTS IN STANDARD RECIPES (arranged alphabetically)	FAVORED INGREDIENTS IN CONVERTED RECIPES
Bacon	Small amounts of smoked yeast (available in health-food stores)

Beef; fatty cuts	*See* page 243.
Bouillon and bouillon cubes	Make your own stock. *See* page 187.
Bread crumbs	Salt-free only. Try making them from my toasted bread.
Butter	Corn oil; no more than 2 tablespoons per recipe. A non-stick skillet, which reduces the need for oil, is preferable.
Cheese	*See* page 248.
Chicken; roasters	Broilers, fryers, cornish hens; *see* page 246.
Consommé; powdered or liquid	Make your own stock. *See* page 187.
Corn starch for thickening	Arrowroot flour
Cottage cheese	Use dry-curd cottage cheese only, no salt added, ½% milkfat. In exceptional cases, mix part-skim ricotta with dry-curd cheese, 1:3 ratio.
Dried dill	Fresh preferred
Egg yolks as thickening agent	Two egg yolks per week are permitted. To thicken sauces, try these alternate methods without eggs: cook until liquid is reduced and naturally thickened; thicken slightly with 2 teaspoons arrowfoot flour dissolved in 2 teaspoons water, and dribble slowly into hot mixture until desired thickness is achieved.
Fish; frozen (unless no fresh fish is available)	Fresh fish preferred (also canned tuna and salmon packed in water, no salt added)
Flour; bleached, for dredging	Unbleached flour. Try mixing half-flour with half-toasted wheat germ, no sugar added.
Gelatin desserts	Make your own. *See* pages 161, 171.
Lamb; fatty cuts	*See* page 243.
Lard	Corn oil; see *Butter* For acceptable margarines see page 252.
Margarine	Corn oil; see *Butter*.
Mayonnaise	Commerical eggless, saltless mayonnaise (available in health-food stores). Try using my salad dressings (pages 184–186).

Meat glaze (Bovril, Maggi)	Make your own brown beef stock with *Diet for Life* ingredients.
M.S.G. (monosodium glutamate)	Totally unnecessary to good cooking; no replacement needed
Mushrooms; canned	Fresh or dried only
Mustard	Mustard prepared without salt.
Olive oil	Use half corn oil and half Italian olive oil.
Parsley; dried	Fresh preferred
Pasta, made with eggs and salt	Pasta made without eggs or salt; *see* page 223.
Peanut oil	Corn oil; see *Butter*
Pepper; black or white	Cayenne pepper
Pork; fatty cuts	*See* pages 243–244.
Safflower oil	Corn oil; see *Butter*
Salt	Minced fresh garlic, minced celery, tangy spices, fresh and dried herbs, as well as aromatic seeds *(see* Chapter 11)
Sugar (white, brown, turbinado, raw, molasses)	Fresh and bottled fruit juices, no sugar added; up to 2 tablespoons honey per recipe; sweet spices *(see* Chapter 11). Use carrots and onions to impart a sweet flavor.
Tabasco	My All-Round Sauce (*See* page 195), using additional cayenne pepper if it is desired
Tomatoes; canned	Diet pack, no salt added
Tomato juice	Diet pack, no salt added
Tomato purée	Diet pack, no salt added
Turkey; frozen, with additives	Fresh only, no additives; young turkeys preferred *(see* page 246)
Veal; fatty cuts	*See* page 243.
Vegetable shortening	Corn oil; see *Butter*
Worcestershire Sauce	Use my All-Round Sauce (*See* page 195).

How to Convert a Meat Dish

Following is a popular basic recipe for braised pot roast. Next to each forbidden ingredient, I've listed the favored ingredient. These additional ingredients are needed to point up flavor:

- Shallots, green pepper, additional garlic—all finely minced
- Augmented quantities of herbs
- Bouquet garni made up of parsley sprigs, bay leaf, and sometimes dill sprigs
- Lime juice, lemon juice, vinegars, wine (red and white)

I've added vinegar to this recipe, but in other meat recipes you might add either lime juice or lemon juice, red or white wine, or combinations.

Use this converted beef recipe as a model for all meat recipe conversions.

POPULAR BASIC RECIPE FOR BRAISED POT ROAST	CONVERTED RECIPE
3 pounds beef, chuck, brisket, or round	3 pounds top or bottom round
2 teaspoons salt	None
¼ teaspoon black pepper	Several dashes cayenne pepper to taste
2 tablespoons peanut oil (or unspecified oil)	2 tablespoons corn oil or combination of corn oil and Italian olive oil
1 large clove garlic, crushed	3-4 large cloves garlic, finely minced—*never* crushed
1 can tomatoes	2 large fresh tomatoes, or equivalent-weight can of tomatoes, no salt or sugar added
1 can beef broth	Equal amount homemade stock *(see recipe for basic stock on page 187)*.
2 small white turnips (not forbidden but doesn't do too much for beef; does more for poultry)	⅓ cup *yellow* turnip. It imparts a more pungent flavor than white. Both kinds of turnip, though, are healthful.
1 teaspoon sugar	⅛ cup apple juice, no sugar added, or 1 teaspoon honey
6 carrots	2 carrots. Carrots are sweet and tend to overpower the dish. They're also high in sodium.
2 medium onions, quartered	1 medium onion, minced. Cooked onions are very sweet.

1 bay leaf	Bouquet garni (see *Added Ingredients* at the close of this recipe)
¼ teaspoon thyme	½ teaspoon each dried thyme and rosemary leaves, crushed, or combination of thyme, rosemary, and sage leaves, crushed
2 ribs celery	Up to 1 rib of celery. Celery is high in sodium and tends to water down flavor.
2 tablespoons of flour for dredging	Optional; less calories without it

Added Ingredients:
2 shallots, minced; 2 tablespoons apple-cider vinegar; ½ green pepper cut into thin slivers; bouquet garni made up of several sprigs parsley tied around a bay leaf with white thread
Optional: 1 tablespoon tomato paste, no salt or sugar added

COOKING HINTS:

1. Always sauté vegetables and garlic in heated oil until wilted or brown. Then add vinegar or wine, and cook for 1 minute. Balance of ingredients are then added.

2. Braise in a slow oven, rather than cooking on top of stove. This reduces meat shrinkage, loss of liquid, and produces a more tender roast.

How to Convert a Chicken Dish

Following are two popular basic recipes for roasting chicken. Recipe #1 produces a bland but palatable bird. Recipe #2, the salt-free way, produces an inedible bird.

TWO POPULAR RECIPES FOR BASIC ROAST CHICKEN	CONVERTED RECIPE
• *Recipe #1*	
3- to 5-pound roasting chicken	3-pound broiler or fryer, skin removed
Butter to brush over bird	Marinade (*see* recipes, pages 105, 132)
Salt, paprika, pepper	All necessary seasonings are included in marinades.
• *Recipe #2*	
3- to 5-pound roasting chicken placed in oven and roasted as is	See conversion for Recipe #1.

COOKING HINTS: Both popular recipes prepare the chicken with skin. I remove the skin *before* cooking. Then marinate in one of my marinades. The results are delicious, diversified, and healthful.

How to Convert a Fish Dish

Following is a popular basic recipe for broiled (or baked) fillet of sole. It's quick and easy.

POPULAR RECIPE FOR BROILED FILLET OF SOLE	CONVERTED RECIPE
1½ pounds fillets of sole	1½ pounds fillets of sole
2-3 tablespoons melted butter or margarine	1-2 tablespoons corn oil
Salt and pepper to taste	2 teaspoons lime juice
	½ teaspoon ground ginger
	4 dashes cayenne pepper
	½ teaspoon dried tarragon leaves, crushed (or 1 teaspoon fresh tarragon, minced)
	1 tablespoon minced celery
	1 large clove garlic, minced
	1 large shallot, minced
	¼-⅓ cup dry vermouth

COOKING HINTS: Rub fish with lime juice and sprinkle with ginger and cayenne. Spread celery, garlic, and shallot in a non-stick skillet and sauté lightly in corn oil. Lay fillets on top of sautéed mixture, sprinkle with herb leaves, and sauté on both sides until lightly browned. Add vermouth and spoon over fish as it cooks for 2 or 3 minutes. (This is a variation of my recipe for *Lobster Taste-Alike*, page 98. See recipe for more explicit directions.)

Forbidden and Favored Ingredients for Baking Cakes, Cookies, and Pies

FORBIDDEN INGREDIENTS IN STANDARD RECIPES (arranged alphabetically)	FAVORED INGREDIENTS IN CONVERTED RECIPES
Baking powder or baking soda	Low-sodium baking powder (available in health-food stores). Use 1½ times the amount baking powder or soda.
Butter	Corn oil, never to exceed ¼ cup per recipe. When replacing butter with oil, it's

	necessary to use more flour than called for in the standard recipe. Occasionally margarine may be used, never to exceed 3 tablespoons per recipe. (*See* page 252.)
Candied fruit	Minced dried fruit, no sugar added
Chocolate	Carob powder, no sugar added
Cocoa	Carob powder, no sugar added
Coconut	Chopped walnuts and almonds
Cream	Non-fat skim milk; evaporated skim milk (¼% milkfat)
Cream; whipped	Skimmed evaporated milk, whipped (¼% milkfat). Frothiness will last up to 10 minutes after serving. Follow directions on can. I prefer beaten egg whites as topping *(see* recipe for *Poached Pears with Spiced Meringue,* page 120).
Eggs; whole, in excess of 1	One whole egg plus 1 egg white. Two egg whites (no yolk) may be substituted for 1 whole egg.
Extracts	Pure only. Imitation extracts have sugar added.
Flour; all-purpose bleached	All-purpose *un*bleached flour
Flour; cake	Unbleached flour sifted 4 times
Jellies	Make your own, or use small amounts of jelly sweetened with honey only.
Milk; evaporated or condensed	*See Cream.*
Milk; whole	*See Cream.*
Mincemeat	*See Candied fruit.*
Nuts	Walnuts and almonds; never more than ¼ cup
Salt, and salt substitutes	Combination of spices, sweet juices, and seeds—not to replace salt, but to provide a more exciting, *new* taste
Sugar (white, brown, turbinado, raw, molasses)	Sweet spices like cinnamon, coriander, nutmeg, allspice, cardamom, ginger, mace, together with naturally sweet fruit juices; also, pure vanilla extract or vanilla beans, and honey.
Yogurt; whole	Low-fat plain yogurt

Forbidden and Favored Ingredients for Baking Bread

FORBIDDEN INGREDIENTS IN STANDARD RECIPES (arranged alphabetically)	FAVORED INGREDIENTS IN CONVERTED RECIPES
Butter	Corn oil (up to 2 tablespoons)
Milk; whole	Non-fat dry milk; non-fat liquid milk; plain low-fat yogurt; buttermilk (no salt added)
Salt	See *Salt* in preceding list.
Sugar	Honey, sweet seeds like coriander and anise, and fruit juices
Water (not a forbidden item, but a partially replaceable one)	Half fruit juices and half water

BAKING HINTS:

1. When a recipe calls for 4-6 whole eggs, it is relying upon the yolks not only for flavor, but to give the cake body. Generally 2 egg whites may be substituted for 1 whole egg. This will hold the batter together.

2. When a recipe calls for more than 2 eggs, use 2 egg whites for each whole egg, or 1 egg yolk and 3 egg whites.

3. When a recipe calls for 1 cup sugar, it's a mighty sweet recipe, and not easily convertible. Try adding date powder, sweet fruit juices, grated orange rind, and chopped dried fruits like raisins, prunes, and dates.

4. When a recipe calls for ½ cup butter or more, it is relying on the butter for flavor. Oil or margarine cannot duplicate the flavor of butter. Such a recipe would not lend itself to a favorable conversion.

5. When fruit juice is used instead of sugar, additional flour is necessary. Specific quantities vary from recipe to recipe. To get the feel of just what amount is right for your conversion, read through the recipes for baked goods in this book (page 189).

9

The Caloric and
Sodium Contents
of Diet for Life Foods

Both excess calories and excess sodium put weight on you. Count the sodium and caloric contents of the following foods before you use them, and you need never exceed your daily caloric allowance (see Chapter 5) or your daily sodium allowance (about 500 milligrams a day). Within the framework of the Diet for Life menu pattern these foods will also help you stay below the daily safety limits for ingested cholesterol (about 160 milligrams) and for fat calories (about 20% of the total caloric intake).

Here's how to get the most from this list:

1. It's divided into two parts: *Diet for Life Foods*; and *Diet for Life Drinks.*

2. So you can use this list trouble-free when you snack, or when you convert recipes or make up your own, calorie and sodium contents are provided in terms of common units (like 4 ounces) or measures with which you are familiar (like teaspoons, tablespoons, and cups).

3. Unless otherwise indicated, food is listed as raw; and meat, fish, and poultry, as edible portions, with visible fat separated. Four ounces of meat, fish, or poultry is roughly equivalent to 3 ounces of the cooked food.

4. UK stands for "unknown," and the term appears only in the sodium column. As a rule of thumb, a UK for fish can be regarded as between 60 and 80; for shellfish, in excess of 100; and for members of the vegetable kingdom, below 10. TB stands for tablespoon, and TS for teaspoon.

5. The sodium contents are provided in milligrams. Numbers have been rounded out to the nearest .5. A 0 means less than .25.

Diet for Life Foods

Food	Serving or measure	Sodium	Calories
Abalone	4 ounces	UK	125
Alewife	4 ounces	UK	142
Apples	1 medium	3.5	75
Apricots	1 medium	.5	18
Apricots, dried	1 medium	1	20
Arrowroot	1 TB	UK	30
Artichokes, French	1 medium	42	48
Artichoke hearts, French	1 medium	13	6.5
Artichokes, Jerusalem	1 small	UK	17
Asparagus stalks	1 medium	0	2
Asparagus spears (cut, 2″ pieces)	¼ cup	2	18
frozen	¼ cup	2	18
Bamboo shoots	4 ounces	UK	35
Bananas	1 medium	6	99
Barley	¼ cup	1.5	200
Barracuda (Pacific)	4 ounces	UK	129
Bass (sea)	4 ounces	78	110
Bass (small-mouth or large-mouth)	4 ounces	UK	119
Bass (striped)	4 ounces	UK	120
Bass (white)	4 ounces	UK	112
Beans:			
green	¼ cup	.5	12
green, frozen	¼ cup	1	12
kidney	¼ cup	1	200
navy	¼ cup	1	16
lima	¼ cup	.5	50
wax (yellow)	¼ cup	.5	12
white marrow	¼ cup	2	160
Bean sprouts:			
mung	¼ cup	1	8
soy	¼ cup	2	18
Beef:			
chuck	4 ounces	74	181
double-bone sirloin	4 ounces	74	181
flank steak	4 ounces	74	163
London broil (hindshank)	4 ounces	74	154
porterhouse (including filet mignon, shell steak, and tailsteak)	4 ounces	74	187
pot roast (foreshank)	4 ounces	74	161

Food	Serving or measure	Sodium	Calories
roast beef (round)	4 ounces	74	155
rump	4 ounces	74	181
short plate	4 ounces	74	187
sirloin steak	4 ounces	74	163
T-bone	4 ounces	74	187
Beets	¼ cup	12	18
Blackberries	¼ cup	1	21
Blueberries	¼ cup	.5	22
Bluefish	4 ounces	85	134
Bread:			
Diet for Life,	slice	2	51
except Norwegian rye	slice	37	77
Broccoli, chopped	¼ cup	5	11
Brussels sprouts, fresh	¼ cup	4.5	21
frozen	¼ cup	11.5	22
Buffalofish	4 ounces	59	129
Burbot	4 ounces	80	89
Butterfish	4 ounces	UK	193
Buttermilk, unsalted	1 cup	120	89
Cabbage, shredded	¼ cup	3	5
Chinese	¼ cup	3	6
Cantaloupe	¼ medium	6	18
Carob	¼ cup	3	110
Carp	4 ounces	57	132
Carrots	1 large	34	20
Cassaba melon	1 medium wedge	12	27
Catfish (freshwater)	4 ounces	69	118
Cauliflower	¼ cup	9	8
Celery	½ rib	12.5	17
Cereals, no sugar or salt added:			
cornflakes	½ cup	1	84
cornmeal, cooked	½ cup	0	30
cream of wheat, cooked	½ cup	0	60
farina, cooked	½ cup	4	68
granola, commercial, no coconut or coconut/palm oils	3 TB	0	110
Maltex, cooked	½ cup	2	71
millet grits, cooked	½ cup	2	60
millet, puffed	½ cup	2	60
oats, rolled, cooked	½ cup	0	77
Ralston, cooked	½ cup	0	77
rice, puffed	½ cup	0	39
wheat, puffed	½ cup	.5	27
wheat, shredded	1 biscuit	4	50
Wheatena, cooked	½ cup	0	103

Food	Serving or measure	Sodium	Calories
wheat germ	1 TB	1	28
Cheese			
acceptables (see page 248)	½ ounce	42-100*	25-50*
cottage cheese, dry-curd skim milk, less than ½% milkfat, no salt added	½ ounce	42	11.5
Cherries	¼ cup	1.5	20
Chestnuts:			
dried	1 ounce	2	36
fresh	1 ounce	1	18
Chives	1 ounce	2	10
Chick peas (garbanzos)	¼ cup	13	188
Chicory	1 leaf	3	1
Chicken, fryers, without skin:			
light meat	4 ounces	62	115
light meat, breast	4 ounces	89	126
dark meat	4 ounces	91	128
dark meat, leg	4 ounces	125	146
Clams, meat only	4 ounces	137	87
Cod	4 ounces	80	89
Corn	1 ear, medium	3	85
popped, no butter or salt added	1 ounce	0	108
Corn oil	1 TB	0	120
Corn starch	1 TB	.5	29
Crab	4 ounces	UK	160
Crabapples	1 average	1	20
Crackers:			
brown rice wafers	1	.5	9
wheat wafers	1	.5	8
Cranberries	¼ cup	.5	13.5
Croaker (Atlantic)	4 ounces	UK	76
Crayfish	4 ounces	UK	82
Cucumbers	1 average	7	20
Currants	¼ cup	1	15
Dates, dried	1	0	21.5
Eggs:	1 medium		
whole		68	87
yolk		13	61
white		55	16
Eggplant	½ medium	8.5	48
Endive	1 leaf	1	2
Escarole	1 leaf	1	1

* (Estimated averages; exact figures unavailable)

Food	Serving or measure	Sodium	Calories
Figs:			
fresh	1 large	1	30
dried	1 large	2	57
Flour:			
all-purpose, unbleached, enriched	¼ cup	0	104
buckwheat	¼ cup	0	87.5
corn	¼ cup	2.5	101.5
gluten	¼ cup	0	108
pastry	¼ cup	0	104
rye, medium	¼ cup	0	100
wheat, whole	¼ cup	2.5	100
soybean, defatted	¼	0	63
Flounder	4 ounces	89	93
Frog legs	4 ounces	UK	83
Garlic	1 clove	1	6
Gelatin, unflavored	1 TB	3.5	34
Gooseberries	¼ cup	0	15
Grapefruit	½ medium	3	75
Grapes	1 medium	0	5
Gray snapper	4 ounces	74	106
Guava	1 average	2	50
Haddock	4 ounces	70	90
Hake	4 ounces	85	85
Halibut	4 ounces	60	144
Ham, fresh boneless	4 ounces	80	144
Herbs	See note at end of list		
Herring:			
Atlantic	4 ounces	74	210
Pacific	4 ounces	85	112
Honey	1 TB	1.5	62
Honeydew melon	1 medium wedge	12	33
Horseradish	1 average	8	87
Huckleberries	½ cup	1	80
Jams and jellies, commercial, sweetened with honey only	1 TB	1	55
Kasha (buckwheat groats)	¼ cup	0	86
Lamb:			
leg	4 ounces	70	148
loin chops and other loin cuts	4 ounces	70	157
rib chops	4 ounces	70	181
shoulder chops	4 ounces	70	169

Food	Serving or measure	Sodium	Calories
Leeks	½ cup	1	10
Lemon	1 medium	0	20
Lentils	¼ cup	2	124
Lettuce	1 leaf	1	1
Lime	1 medium	0	20
Lobster:			
Atlantic	4 ounces	UK	104
spiny	4 ounces	UK	82
Loganberries	¼ cup	0	22.5
Mackerel:			
Atlantic	4 ounces	60	204
Pacific	4 ounces	UK	182
Macaroni, no salt added	2 ounces	0	210
Mango	1 medium	4	133
Matzoh:			
Passover	1	0	112
thins	1	9.5	90
Mayonnaise:			
commercial, eggless, low-sodium	1 TB	6	92
Melba toast:			
commercial, low-sodium	1	1.5	15
Milk:			
evaporated, skim	½ cup	128	90
non-fat, dry	1 TB	43	30
non-fat, liquid	1 cup	128	90
Mullet	4 ounces	93	167
Mushrooms	1 large	1.5	3
Mussels, meat only	4 ounces	320	109
Mustard greens	1 cup	8	30
Nectarines	1 medium	4	40
Okra	1 pod	0	1.5
Onion	1 medium	6	26
Orange	1 medium	2	70
Oysters, meat only:			
Eastern	4 ounces	84	75
Pacific and Western	4 ounces	UK	104
Papaya	1 medium	6	43
Peaches	1 average	2	51
Pears	1 average	2	60
Peas:			
shelled	¼ cup	5	28
split, dried	¼ cup	12.5	172

Food	Serving or measure	Sodium	Calories
Pepper, green	1 average	1	16
Perch:			
white	4 ounces	UK	134
yellow	4 ounces	UK	135
Persimmons	1 average	5	95
Pike	4 ounces	58	106
Pineapple:			
canned, no sugar added; cubes	½ cup	0	37.5
fresh	½" slice	0	35
Plums	1 average	.5	29
Pollock	4 ounces	55	109
Pomegranate	1 average	3	75
Popcorn, unpopped	1 TB	1	76
popped: see Corn			
Porgy	4 ounces	72	129
Pork, picnic	4 ounces	70	155
Potatoes:			
sweet	1 medium	12	183
white	1 medium	11	110
Prunes	1 small	.5	18
Pumpkin	1 cup	2	66
Quince	1 average	3	40
Rabbit	4 ounces	53	140
Radish	1 average	3	2
Raisins, seedless	1 TB	3	60
Raspberries:			
black	¼ cup	0	21
red	¼ cup	0	18
Redfish (ocean perch)	4 ounces	77	106
Rhubarb, diced	¼ cup	2	20
Rice:			
brown	¼ cup	1	212
instant	¼ cup	0	214
white, enriched	¼ cup	0	213
Rockfish	4 ounces	68	113
Safflower oil	1 TB	0	125
Salad dressing, Diet for Life	1 TB	1	62
Salmon:			
canned, in water, no salt added	4 ounces	95	221
fresh, Atlantic	4 ounces	UK	248
fresh, pink (humpback)	4 ounces	73	136
Scallions	1 average	1	5
Scallops	4 ounces	UK	90

Food	Serving or measure	Sodium	Calories
Scrod	4 ounces	89	93
Scup	4 ounces	72	109
Sea bass: see *Bass*			
Shad	4 ounces	62	195
Shallots	1	1.5	8.5
Shrimp	4 ounces	159	104
Skate	4 ounces	UK	110
Smelts	4 ounces	UK	131
Snails	4 ounces	UK	103
Sole	4 ounces	89	93
Soursop	4 ounces	16	74
Sprouts:			
mung	¼ cup	1	10
soy	¼ cup	1	12
Spaghetti, no salt added	¼ cup	1	96
Spices	*See note at end of list.*		
Spinach	¼ cup	82.5	22.5
Squash:			
summer	¼ cup	0	22.5
winter	¼ cup	0	15
Squid	4 ounces	UK	96
Sturgeon	4 ounces	UK	167
Swordfish	4 ounces	90	140
Tangerines	1 average	16	35
Tile fish	4 ounces	UK	92
Tofu	4 ounces	8	158
Tomatoes:			
canned, no salt added	½ cup	15	25
fresh	1 average	3	30
Tomato paste, no salt added	1 TB	9	18
Tomato purée, no salt added	1 TB	1.5	1
Trout:			
brook	4 ounces	UK	115
lake	4 ounces	UK	160
Tuna:			
canned, in water, no salt added	4 ounces	60	122
fresh, bluefin	4 ounces	UK	167
fresh, yellowfin	4 ounces	42	154
Turkey:			
mature, dark meat	4 ounces	81	145
mature, white meat	4 ounces	51	130
young, dark meat	4 ounces	81	127
young, white meat	4 ounces	51	123
Turnip greens, cooked	½ cup	10	22
Turnip, yellow, cooked	½ cup	5	25

Food	Serving or measure	Sodium	Calories
Veal:			
leg	4 ounces	90	149
loin chops and other loin cuts	4 ounces	90	178
round and rump	4 ounces	90	160
shoulder chops and chuck	4 ounces	90	160
Venison	4 ounces	UK	112
Vinegar:			
cider or distilled	1 TB	0	2
red-wine	1 TB	4	2
white-wine	1 TB	5	2
Walnuts	1 medium	0	26
Water chestnuts	1 average	1	5
Watercress	1 bunch	44	16.5
Watermelon	1 thick slice	0	13
Weakfish	4 ounces	86	108
Wheat germ	1 ounce	1	110
Wreckfish	4 ounces	UK	130
Yams	1 average	UK	200
Yeast, compressed	1 TB	.5	20
Yellowtail	4 ounces	UK	156
Yogurt, skim-milk	1 cup	129	115
Zucchini	¼ cup	1.5	7.5

Diet for Life Drinks

Drink	Serving or measure	Sodium	Calories
Apple cider	½ cup	1	62
Apple juice	½ cup	6	62
Apricot juice	½ cup	4	51
Cranberry juice, unsweetened	½ cup	3	90
Coffee taste-alikes:			
Cafix (no caffeine)	1 TS	UK	7
Nescafé, dry instant	1 TS	1	0
Sanka, dry instant	1 TS	UK	0
Grape juice	½ cup	4	85
Grapefruit juice	½ cup	2	65
Lemon juice	½ cup	2	32
Orange juice	½ cup	2.5	54
Perrier mineral water	½ cup	UK	0
Pineapple juice	½ cup	.5	60
Prune juice	½ cup	2	85

Food	Serving or measure	Sodium	Calories
Tangerine juice	½ cup	2	47
Tomato juice:			
canned, no salt added	½ cup	6	28
fresh	½ cup	6	25
Wine:			
dry red	4 ounces	8	84
dry white	4 ounces	11	84
sherry (cooking)	1 TB	2.5	22
sweet	4 ounces	11	144

Notes on the Caloric and Sodium Contents of Herbs and Spices

Since most herbs and spices are used in very small amounts (a dash is less than ⅛ of a teaspoon), you may regard their caloric and sodium contributions as zero, with the following exceptions:

1. Dried parsley contains 39 milligrams of sodium per teaspoon. The sodium content of fresh parsley is about 2 milligrams a garnish.

2. The sodium content of dried herbs in general is higher than their fresh counterparts. As a rule of thumb, figure 10 milligrams of sodium per teaspoon of dried herbs.

3. Chile con carne *seasoning,* which is a favored Diet for Life food, contains no salt and has about 1 milligram of sodium per teaspoon. Chile con carne *powder,* on the other hand, has about 57 milligrams.

4. Avoid garlic salt (more than 800 milligrams of sodium per teaspoon), celery salt (about 840 milligrams), and celery flakes (about 115 milligrams).

5. Pure extracts are virtually sodium free; and since the alcohol evaporates on baking, are almost calorie-free in small quantities as well. Avoid extracts with sugar added.

PART THREE

Eating Healthfully for the Rest of Your Life

10

Everything You Should Know About Starches, Grains, Breads, Pasta, Seeds, Sprouts, Beans, Peas, Lentils, Nuts, Fructose, Carob, Honey, and Fiber

We recommend potatoes.

"Potatoes!" shocked dieters shriek. "How can you recommend potatoes! They're a starch food! They put weight on you!"

Potato-shunning is part of the nation's weight-control folklore.

Yet a five-ounce potato contains only 110 calories. It has no cholesterol and virtually no fat, is rich in vitamins (particularly C and B_3) and minerals (including potassium and iron), and has as much fiber as bean sprouts. It contains—and here's the biggest surprise of all—a significant amount of protein.

Some food experts claim that potatoes are so well-balanced nutritionally that an adult can live on them and very little else. Indeed, much of the population of Ireland in the last century did survive on them almost exclusively. It was the failure of the potato crops which triggered the great wave of Irish emigration to the United States.

Yes, the potato is starchy, but—

Starches Are Good for You

Starches are complex carbohydrates. Sugar (sucrose) is a simple carbohydrate. Carbohydrates, both simple and complex, are the body's main source of energy. Digested easily, they are broken down by the body's chemistry into one of the simplest of all sugars, glucose. Carried in the bloodstream, glucose fuels the brain, the muscles, and all the cells of the body. Your body has no need for sucrose for fuel so long as sufficient amounts of complex carbohydrates are included in your diet.

Starches are not fattening. Like all carbohydrates, they contribute the same four calories a gram as proteins, far less than the nine calories contributed by fats. Starchy foods—which include nutrient-rich fruits, vegetables, grains, legumes, nuts, seeds, pasta, and breads —are preferred to sucrose, which supplies only empty calories. Like the potato, carbohydrate foods often contain astonishing quantities of proteins (some beans contain almost as much as meat), an ample supply of many vitamins and minerals, and sufficient fiber to meet your body's requirements.

Metabolized slowly, starches put no strain on the body's chemistry. On the other hand, refined sugar is metabolized rapidly, causing sudden surges and precipitate drops in blood-sugar (glucose) levels which can disturb the entire chemical balance of the body. This, in turn, over long periods of time, can open pathways to degenerative diseases, including heart attack. Refined sugar is banned from the Diet for Life not only because it is an empty-calorie food, but also because it is associated with cardiovascular risk. To the healthy person, there is no risk of any kind from starchy foods when consumed as part of a balanced diet.

Here is a review of the kinds of starch foods in the Diet for Life, including some that contain acceptable sugars.

The Fabulous Grains

Wheat and rye. In wheat, as in all grains, the kernel (the whole grain) consists of three parts: the endosperm, which provides the nutrients for the growing seedling, is high in starch and protein; the germ, which is the nutrient source for the plant's first roots and leaves, is rich in polyunsaturated fats, protein, vitamins B_1 and E, and iron; and the bran, which is the grain's protective covering, is composed almost entirely of fiber. The whole grain is more nutritious than any of its parts.

For breakfast, I serve wheat in the form of commercial cereals with no salt or sugar added. Our favorite packaged cold wheat cereals are shredded wheat and puffed wheat (both of which are made from the whole grain). Our favorite packaged hot wheat cereals are cream of wheat, which is enriched farina (the purified endosperm of certain kinds of hard wheat); Wheatena, which is a toasted and processed whole-grain product; and cracked wheat made from whole kernels (I also blend cracked wheat into some of my breads).

Bulgur, a pre-cooked cracked wheat with a nutty taste, has yet to catch our fancy; besides the only commercial sources I know contain salt.

I use wheat germ to sprinkle on other cereals to provide crunchiness, and as an ingredient in my own granolas. (Most commercial granolas are to be avoided since they contain salt, sugar, molasses, preservatives, and coconut, which is high in saturated fats. Unsweetened and unsalted Muesli is a nutritionally acceptable granola-type product, but it doesn't pass our taste test.)

I use wheat flour in my bread, rolls, pies, cakes, cookies, breadings, and stuffings. I use rye, which matches wheat nutritionally, solely as a bread flour. (There's a great deal more information on wheat and rye flours beginning on page 220.)

Rice loses much of its nutritional value when the brown hull and bran layers (rich sources of Vitamin B_1 and fiber) are removed by the milling process to produce the more familiar white rice. I don't use long-grain brown rice because it cooks into a gooey mess. I prefer the short-grain variety distinctively flecked with green. The kernels cook up moist and tender, with only the slightest tendency to stick together.

I like my rice kernels to be rich, plump individuals, and they always emerge that way when I use enriched white rich. It's a notch below brown rice in nutritional value, but it's more easily digested and more compatible gastronomically with a wide variety of my dishes. Enriched converted rice and instant or minute rice also rate B+ nutritionally, but are at the bottom of the class in taste and texture.

Oats. I use oats, properly gussied up, for a steaming-hot energy booster on a frigid winter's morning; as an uncooked ingredient in a granola mix; and as the heart and soul of my mouth-watering cookies. Oats are particularly valuable as a breakfast food, because, high in protein as well as complex carbohydrates, they stick with you during that long hiatus to lunch, and help you spurn the temptations of the mid-morning coffee break.

Whole-grain rolled oats get my nod. Rolling is the least nutritionally damaging of all methods of oat processing, and does little to alter the full-flavored sweetness and hearty texture of this versatile cereal. With each spoonful you'll be downing old-fashioned taste goodness, plus nine minerals, seven vitamins of the B-complex group, and vitamins C and E.

Barley and millet. Unfortunately, whole-grain barley is rare. If you can find it, snap it up. If not, settle for pearl barley, an attractively polished pearly grain from which the hull and bran (with their fiber and B vitamins) have been removed. Still, it offers a plethora of minerals and not an insignificant quantity of vitamin B_3. This moist, sweet, nut-flavored grain makes a superb rice or potato replacement, and is superb in soups.

Millet can be obtained in the nutritious whole grain; but, despite its rising popularity among health aficionados, it's too bland to merit inclusion among my recipes. My only use for this grain is as a puffed breakfast cereal (no sugar or salt added) served cold with non-fat milk. If you have an acid-stomach problem, though, you may want to add millet to your menus. It's alkaline (most grains are acidic), and it can be put to as many culinary uses as barley.

Corn. What rice is to the millions of Asiatics, corn (the rest of the world calls it maize) was to the American Indians. They thrived on it—toasting it, boiling it, drying it, and making flat cakes from the ground corn which sustained them through long winters. It is a superb food, as laden with vitamins and minerals as oats or wheat, and particularly high in vitamin A, phosphorus, and potassium.

Gourmet cuisine shuns it, although open-minded gastronomes delight in some Italian corn dishes. I serve corn, which I de-cob myself, as a side dish; I use corn flour in baking; and some of our breakfasts include puffed corn (no sugar or salt added). We snack on home-made popcorn with little more than a soupçon of oil, and not a grain of salt. Delicious!

Buckwheat is not a wheat at all. It's not even a grain. It's the *seed* of an herb. (A grain is the seed of a cereal grass.) But it looks like a grain, it cooks like a grain, it grinds to flour like a grain, and its nutritional profile resembles a grain's.

I use the flour in griddle cakes (it would be un-American not to); and I blend other flours with buckwheat to create delectable breads and rolls. The toasted whole grain called kasha has long been an East European favorite, and it's one of ours. Cooked the only way it should be (it can be a disaster if it's not; see my recipe on page 142), it's featured on my table as a palate-pleasing alternate to potatoes, rice, and barley.

Grain Foods: Breads and Rolls

Bread was once called "the staff of life." In the hands of our commercial breadmakers, however, it's not. Dr. Jean Mayer, former nutrition consultant to the White House, referred to slices of store-bought bread as "edible napkins." My only cavil with his judgment is the word "edible."

But you can bring back bread's traditional appeal. You can make breads zesty with the wholesomeness of vital nutrients, and heartily crusted, textured, and flavored with—I have no other word for it—*breadiness.* All you have to do is follow my recipes. You'll transform dough once more into the staff of life—while you're having the time of your life!

It's fun, true excitement, to make a bread. You're an artist, molding and shaping. You're a creator, bringing life to the inanimate—for dough rises, bubbles, and grows with a life of its own. You're an esthete luxuriating in the feel of the dough's texture, the scents of its perfumes. And you're a hard-nosed bookkeeper with a grin on your face, because you know "baking it yourself" looks great on the bottom line. There's no more satisfying aroma than that of bread baking in the oven. There's no more satisfying food than a freshly baked loaf.

As a bread-maker, you won't be alone. Eighty percent of the flour currently sold to U.S.A. consumers goes into bread; and the number of the nation's breadmakers is swelling so rapidly that one giant mill recently launched an unprecedented "Bread Flour." Bread-making is in. (But Bread Flour is out of my recipes. In my test run, it had none of claimed dough-rising properties; and it's higher in sodium than unbleached flour.)

Opt for stone-ground flours, even though the price tags are high. In stone-grinding, whole grains are placed between millstones no more than a grain's breadth apart, and gently reduced to flour. The delicate structures of the nutrients, which are crushed under massive rolling mills in standard grinding processes, remain intact; and the highly polyunsaturated oils and vitamin E-rich germ are distributed evenly throughout the flour. You're more likely to find stone-ground flour in health-food stores than in supermarkets, but it's worth the detour if a bread with the old-fashioned flavor and texture is your heart's desire.

Here is the core information on the kind of flours I use in the Diet for Life. They make breads that contribute only about 55 calories a slice. (Whenever, in the following passages, I refer to bread-making, read roll-making as well. Any of my bread recipes can easily be converted to a roll recipe.)

Whole-wheat flour, as the name connotes, is milled from the whole grain. Toasted whole-wheat bread has a delicious aroma unmatched by any other toasted bread. A rough variant of whole-wheat flour is Graham flour, named after the pre-Civil War health-food pioneer Sylvester Graham, who invented Graham crackers. The supermarket product labeled "Whole Wheat Flour [graham]" is finely ground, and not true Graham with a capital G. If you can find true Graham flour—and you won't find it easily—you'll be able to bake a bread as rare as it is packed with chewing goodness.

Unbleached enriched all-purpose wheat flour. Unbleached means no chemical, such as chlorine dioxide, has been added to remove the yellowish color which wheat flour takes on at the end of the milling process. Bleaching destroys nutrients, texture, and taste. If the flour is permitted to stand eight to 12 weeks after milling, the yellow color disappears naturally, and the result is unbleached flour.

"Enriched" means that certain vitamins and minerals are added to the milled flour in accordance with federal and state laws to restore in large part the nutrients lost in the milling process. In that process the bran is removed to make a smoother-textured flour; and the wheat germ is extracted because its high oil content decreases shelf life. Yet, except for its lack of fiber, enriched unbleached flour does not compare unfavorably with whole-wheat flour in health values, and it has far greater versatility in the kitchen.

"All-purpose" means that the flour can be used for yeast breads and cakes, or for pastries, quickbreads, nutbreads, muffins, pancakes, waffles, cookies, and cakes made with baking powder or baking soda. All-purpose flour is composed of a mixture of hard wheat, suitable for yeast breads and cakes, and soft wheat, suitable for pastries. The combination lends itself to a variety of breads of fascinating tastes and textures.

Gluten flour is hard wheat flour from which most of the starch has been removed, and is consequently high in proteins. One of the proteins is gluten, one of nature's wonders. It's an elastic adhesive which holds the dough together, and yet lets the dough rise as it's pushed upward by the pressure of the carbon dioxide gas generated by the yeast. Without sufficient gluten, which is present in substantial amounts in all hard wheats, bread dough cannot rise. (Soft wheat—pastry flour—must be leavened by baking powder or baking soda.) In gluten flour the concentration of gluten is high. When I use large amounts of dark flours (low in gluten), I mix in gluten flour to produce high-rising dough and light loaves.

Gluten bread, because of its high protein content, is found frequently in the diets of diabetics. Neither Harold nor I regards it as an unqualified delight.

Rye flour. There are four kinds. *Pumpernickel flour* is made from the whole grain, and it produces a dense, nutty-flavored, dark brown bread which needs no artificial coloring (commercial pumpernickel does). *Dark rye flour* is milled from the whole grain minus some of the bran and starch. *Medium rye flour* contains no bran, and is light gray in color. And then there is *light rye flour,* which is heavily processed. In these four varieties, as the brownness of the flour fades, so does the flavor and texture.

Pumpernickel flour is next to impossible to find. (A pumpernickel flour offered by one of Manhattan's elite gourmet shops is a mixture of dark rye and whole-wheat flours.) Dark and light rye flours are difficult to locate, as well, but some gourmet shops carry them. Forget about light rye flour, but if you can find dark rye flour, grab it. It will bake into a true rye-tasting, rye-textured loaf. Medium rye flour is available in your supermarket, and even the most ardent rye bread lovers can't fault it. Unlike white flours, dark flours are not required by federal and state laws to be enriched; but medium rye flour is on a par nutritionally with enriched wheat flours.

Rye flours, which have little gluten, rise with difficulty, and tend to form dense, heavy loaves. My rye breads are light and airy because I mix limited amounts of rye flour with high-gluten flours. Rye flour, I've discovered, included in any salt-free bread, helps eliminate the sense of salt deprivation.

My innovative hybrid mixes are an array of inventive combinations of flours and other ingredients used to produce a shelf of new bread favorites. My four-flour bread unconventionally calls for rye, whole-wheat, unbleached, and gluten flours. I daringly inject buckwheat flour into many of my mixes to heighten flavor. I make imaginative use in my breads of one or more of the following flavor-stimulators: herbs and seeds, apple juice and date powder, and even chicken stock. But I don't forget the good old standbys: cracked wheat in some of my mixes to add crunchiness and toastiness; and cornmeal sprinkled on my baking pans to impart that irresistible crackle to the bottom crust of my loaves.

I find bread-making the most fulfilling of all the delights of the kitchen because of its infinite creative possibilities. You will, too.

Pasta Power

It's not pasta that pops your buttons; it's what you put *on* the pasta: cheese, prosciutto, cream, ham, bacon, beef, anchovies, eggs, salt, olive oil, sausage, mortadella, nuts, olives, veal, pork, salt pork, soup, sauces, ground meat, butter . . . The right kind of pasta by itself is only marginally more caloric than Diet for Life breads. Commercial macaroni has about 100 calories an ounce; Diet for Life bread, about 90.

There are two basic types of pasta:

North Italian, or Bolognese, pasta is made from flour, water, eggs, and sometimes olive oil. You'll know it's a North Italian pasta if it bears such names as lasagne, vermicelli, fettucine, ravioli, tagliatelle, cappelletti, agnolotti, or just plain noodles. If you're watching your cholesterol (eggs) and fats (olive oil), as you should on the Diet for Life, put North Italian pasta on your risk list.

Southern, or Neapolitan, pasta, on the other hand, is made only from flour and water. You can identify it by such names as spaghetti, capelli d'angelo, macaroni, linguine, rigatoni, shells, and elbows.

And—*bravissimo!*—no true pasta is made with salt.

Colored pastas are produced by mixing finely ground vegetables into the dough before it is rolled out into sheets. Spinach turns the dough into *pasta verde,* and beets or tomatoes turn it into *pasta rosa.* Every region of Italy shapes its pasta in a distinctive style. In

Bologna it's flat ribbons, in Rome long strips, and in Sicily spirals. You can find pasta in strands as thin as an angel's hair, and in short, stubby cylinders like sections of pipe; in leaves as finely textured as napoleon pastry, and in coarse, doughy, misshapen balls. No other food comes in so many shapes and forms. In a shop in Rome, Harold and I counted about 200 different varieties of pasta.

The American-made pasta we prefer is produced from a strain of red-berried hard durum wheat, grown mostly in North Dakota and Manitoba, Canada. The yellow-white, pasta-colored flour called semolina is in the same nutritional class as enriched, unbleached all-purpose flour. Unless pastas made with other than semolina flour are labeled enriched, pass them by.

You can make your own pasta. I don't. Two reasons: in Manhattan, you can buy excellent freshly made pasta (I expect you can in other urban centers, too); and packaged pastas, particularly those carried by health-food stores, rate 8 out of 10 on our taste meter.

I cook my pasta as the Italians do, *al dente,* slightly resistant to the bite, yet yielding gracefully. According to the legend, when the Bishop of Naples tasted the first pasta cooked in the Western world, he exclaimed, *"Ma caroni!"*—"My little darlings!" And, the legend continues, ever since, macaroni has been the synonym for pasta. Cooked with loving care, and bathed with my sauces, your pasta can become welcome little darlings on those meatless, poultryless, and fishless nights.

The Sensational Seeds: Sprouts, Legumes (Beans, Peas, and Lentils), and Nuts

Grains are one kind of seeds. Seeds, like grains, are natural nutritional storehouses. One structural difference between the two: in seeds, the starch endosperm is less prominent, so seeds are higher in protein than grains (best example: beans) and higher in fat (best example: nuts).

Since the '60s seeds have created a sensation among health-conscious Americans. Here is why and how I use some of them in the Diet for Life, and why I don't use others.

The health-food store seeds were thrust into prominence by the phenomenal expansion of the health-food stores within the last generation. (Health food is now a multi-billion-dollar, earth-girdling industry. One of our sons discovered a health-food store on a sparsely populated island in the Pacific.) Our criticism of health-food store seeds follows.

Raw unsalted sunflower seeds make sensible snacks if you like them. We don't. Without salt, raw pumpkin seeds are our idea of nothing to chew. (But roasted and salted, they become *pepitas,* a Mexican favorite for centuries.) Raw flax seeds fail our taste test, too. Mixed in granolas, where their tastes are diluted by other ingredients, all three are acceptable (they do add crunchiness). But we draw the line at raw alfalfa seeds under any conditions; we can't stand the taste (horses like it, though).

Another drawback: although these seeds are highly nutritious, they *are* fatty (fats contribute 76% of calories in sunflower seeds, for example), and when you swallow a handful you're taking in a big glob of fat, albeit mostly polyunsaturated fat.

The spice seeds. There's another group of seeds that have long been prized by chefs and bakers from the steppes of Asia to the delis of New York. As bursting with healthful nutrients as health-food store seeds, and not as fatty, they're aromatic, flavorful, and marry happily with the ingredients of a great variety of doughs and dishes. Raw or toasted, and used with finesse, they put their signatures on many culinary delights. How could you possibly recognize Jewish rye bread if it didn't have caraway seeds? Caraway, as well as other spice seeds like poppy, fennel, and coriander, are described in the following chapter.

There's one spice seed that has been adopted by the health-food industry with extraordinary success; and that's sesame. Nutty, crunchy, nutritious, and eminently cookable, it deserves its success—as a *seed.* But as an oleaginous paste, tahini, it's a gastronomic nightmare. I use sesame seeds in baking, and to enliven vegetables and salads. The ground seeds mixed with honey make a pleasant halvah-like dessert, but not for calorie-counters or fat-watchers.

Sprouts. They're great! Sprouts are far more nutritious than the seeds from which they are germinated. Fresh as springtime, bursting with the tender flavor of greens, succulent and crunchy, they perk up salads and sandwiches, and make scrumptious snacks alone or used in dips. They even bring a new enchantment to such old favorites as omelettes and braised vegetables. And sautéed with tofu, they can bring the Orient right into your kitchen.

We prefer young mung bean sprouts for their sturdy crunchiness and beany flavor (*caution:* they age badly). Alfalfa sprouts, as they emerge from their plastic packaging, are too often flaccid and bland. But you can grow alfalfa sprouts at home—as well as you can grow many others, including chia, wheatberry, wheat grass, soy, and lentil. But unless you have a green thumb (we don't), you'll end up with patches of sickly swamps on your windowsill. Freshly plucked sprouts, though, are a taste thrill, and it's worth the effort to learn the knack of growing them.

Beans. Kidney beans, pinto beans, calico beans, green beans, yellow beans, red beans—there are dozens of varieties of beans available to the sophisticated seed shopper, and we welcome all of them on our table enthusiastically, except one. We don't like soybeans. Despite their undisputed virtues—twice as much protein as meat or fish, rich in lecithin and polyunsaturated fats—we simply can't stand the taste. There are some foods that no amount of kitchen wizardry can transform into the palatable, and soybeans are close to the top of the list. Soya flour and soya milk, which is made from soya flour, are equally as distasteful to us. (Soya flour is made from lightly toasted beans; soy flour from raw beans.)

Because of its high protein content, the soybean has become the base of a family of imitation-meat products, which derive almost all their flavor from salt. When it comes to pinch-hitting for a beef stroganoff, soybean simulates aren't even in the league. And if you're keeping fats down to 20% of your total caloric intake, as you should, think about this: even though most of their fat is polyun-saturated, mature raw, dry soy seeds are fattier than an equivalent amount of lean sirloin.

One derivative of the soybean, though, is favored in my kitchen. Soybean curd, or tofu. It has little more than one gram of fat per ounce, is an excellent source of protein (the protein to carbohydrate ratio is about 2:1), and is jam-packed with all sorts of nutritional necessities.

But even though it's high in protein, don't expect meatiness from tofu. And don't expect taste or biteyness from the mushy, pallid slabs as they come from the market. Tofu requires doctoring. Cod-dled with inventive sauces and accompanied by flavorsome and firm-textured vegetables, this insipid curd can become an exciting dining experience. It also makes—and here's an eyebrow-raiser—an excellent filling for an omelette (page 102).

Peas and lentils, like beans, are legumes, so named because they come from pod-bearing plants called *leguminosae.* They resemble beans in nutritional values: high in protein, and well stocked with vitamins and minerals.

One class of peas, sweet peas, makes a sprightly vegetable dish. Another class, field peas, are dried into split peas, which in my kitchen are transformed into hearty soups and side dishes. Snow peas—the pod, not the dwarf peas, is the *pièce de résistance* here—add an exotic crunchiness to some of my recipes.

I use the American brown lentils (red or orange ones come from the Middle East) much as I do split peas.

Nuts. Most nuts are too high in saturated fats to qualify for the Diet for Life. Paradoxically, of the few that do, two—walnuts and almonds—cannot be classified as carbohydrate foods. They're actu-ally fatty foods. Walnuts are 64% fat, almonds 54%. But both find a place because the fats in each are 96% polyunsaturated, the highest in any natural food; and because walnuts contain a large quantity of the essential fatty acid called arichidonic, which helps fight cardiovascular diseases.

Both nuts contribute a large number of calories (32 from a walnut, 28 from an almond), so I use them sparingly in cakes, desserts, and salads; with raisins as snacks; and, after a particularly low-fat meal, as mini-desserts combined with a variety of fresh and dried fruits.

There are two other favored nuts in the Diet for Life. Water chestnuts have virtually no fat. I employ them in some of my recipes not for taste (they have none), but for their superlative crunchiness. Chestnuts have a negligible fat content; roast to a taste thrill, and purée to become the launching pads for flights of dessert fancies.

If you're a pecan lover—and who isn't!—proceed with caution. The fat is 95% polyunsaturated, which is good; but the nut is a scary 74% fat, and a single nut contains 42 calories.

Simple Sugars You Can Enjoy without Fear

When is a sugar not an empty calorie? When it's packaged with an abundance of vital nutrients. These packages are called fruits, vegetables, milk (and some derivatives), carob, and honey. All in all, they contain 21 varieties of natural sugars, of which sucrose is one. None of these sugars in the natural state has been indicted by medical research as a potential causative agent for any degenerative diseases. If your carbohydrate metabolism is normal, you can enjoy these natural sweeteners without fear.

And that includes the fear of getting fat. Fruits and vegetables, essentially starchy foods, are low in calories (80 for an apple; 30 for a carrot), and pack enough bulk and water to give you that satisfying stomach-filling feeling. High-bulk grapefruit (75 calories a half) has long been a standard item on weight-reducing diets.

Sun-ripened fruits are sensual delights. But, alas, we're city dwellers; and most fruits, plucked unripe, plastic-packaged, and shipped from up to several thousand miles away, arrive tired, immature, and pulpy, *sans* sweetness and flavor. Never in the last 10 years have Harold and I found a strawberry we liked in the New York market. Apples are edible in season, but pears, peaches, and plums more often than not are consigned to the cooking pot, and melons only hint at their potential lusciousness. There's one exception to the monotony of non-fruit in the Big Apple. For one brief shining week or so in the late spring, cherries hereabouts are superb; and ever so slightly chilled, they become an addictive dessert (low-calorie too!).

We slake our passion for fresh fruit by cutting up the flesh of many fruits into salads, coaxing a synergism of colors, textures, and tastes to create a whole greater than the sum of its parts.

Vegetables are another matter. Our Korean markets, so-called because they are enterprises operated by Korean families, rush in fresh produce from not-too-distant farms. If we hand-pick with care—a minimum of plastic packaging here—we can fill our shopping bags with vegetables as close to garden-fresh as a city dweller can hope for. Salad greens, too, are succulent and crisp (and the lowest in calories of all carbohydrates, as well as brimming with vitamins and minerals). But nothing is quite like your own-grown greens and vegetables; and when Harold, who is mad for radishes, plucked one from his hostess's garden in the Salt Lake Valley, he said, "I've never tasted a radish before."

Freshly squeezed fruit juices can be either wonderful or awful, depending on the quality of the fruits from which they're squeezed; and few fresh juices here in town are worth the bother. In our household, bottled apple juice and soft apple cider (both about 124 calories an 8-ounce glass) are the preferred fruit drinks. Careful: Carrot juice is a favorite of health-food fans, but it contains 268 milligrams of sodium per cup.

Dried fruits, with their extremely high concentration of sugars, can be almost as hazardous to dental health as refined sugars. But dried fruits are almost as nutritious as the fresh; and their sugars, like those of fresh fruits, are not empty calories. Used in moderation, these tart-and-sweet delights make energy-packed snacks eaten raw, and they cook into sweet-tooth-soothing desserts. A snatch of raisins (35 calories) during afternoon doldrums can stimulate your waning get-up-and-go, and lift your spirits. I use dried date powder as a sweetener.

Fructose, fruit sugar, is the dominant sugar in both fruits and vegetables. In those natural packages it's a nutritious and delightful source of energy. But as a refined sugar, it's as likely to hasten tooth decay as any other refined sugar. Its association with degenerative diseases is unproven; and since it's metabolized more slowly than sucrose, it may be of some benefit to some diabetics.

In certain foods and beverages, and within prescribed temperature limits, refined fructose is sweeter than sucrose; so the sweets lover may be inclined to spoon in less fructose than sucrose and conserve a few calories. But refined fructose has no special weight-reducing properties; and in 1979 the U.S. Postal Service moved against mail-order houses whose advertisements claimed a fructose diet would result in an automatic weight loss. (The Fabulous Fructose Diet is, in actuality, a high-fat diet.)

In *non-fat milk* (any other kind is *verboten*), the carbohydrate calories (about 100 to an 8-ounce glass) come mostly from lactose, milk sugar. Milk, with its potentially lethal load of fat removed, in whole or in great part, remains a treasure house of proteins, vitamins, and minerals (especially calcium). Lactose is also present in low-fat yogurt, low-fat cheeses, and buttermilk (which, despite its name, is low in fat). I utilize the natural sweetness of non-fat milk in many of my dishes and in my Frothy Fruit Milkshake (see page 140). Low-fat milk derivatives are far from sweet, but if you like them, remember: lactose contributes to the flavor.

Carob, one of the more felicitous discoveries of the health movement of the '60s, is a chocolate-look-alike sweetener with a delicate and chocolaty underflavor. But chocolate lovers, be warned: the dominant flavor is distinctly its own, more date-like than anything else.

Carob powder is made from the roasted pods of the carob tree (the pods have been known for ages as Saint-John's-bread). The powder is iron- and fiber-rich, contains substantial amounts of other minerals and proteins, and is very, very sweet (about 46% natural sugars). I use carob in puddings, cakes, and in milk drinks.

Honey in some cultures is regarded as the perfect food. It is composed of 31% glucose, 38% fructose, and a little over 1% sucrose in an aromatic amalgam of protein *plus* iron, copper, manganese, potassium, sodium, calcium, magnesium, and other vital elements, *plus* ample quantities of B vitamins and vitamin C, *plus* nine out of 10 amino acids essential to healthful human nutrition. (Amino acids are the building blocks from which the proteins in our body are made.)

There is some scientific evidence to indicate that honey has antibacterial properties. Certainly, there are no storage problems with honey. It remains fresh for years without refrigeration or preservatives, and with little or no deterioration of vitamin values. Folklore medicine has long ascribed a litany of cures to honey, ranging from the soothing of sore throats to the improvement of stomach disorders. On the other hand, modern medical science has indicted honey, along with other high-sugar products, as a dental hazard.

Honey not only sweetens beautifully (it's twice as effective as sucrose), but it brings a variety of enchanting flavors to my dishes. No two kinds of honey taste alike, and there are dozens of kinds to savor. Honey-tasting is a delightful adventure to us, and even though we've settled on our favorites, we're still on the lookout for new labels and the new tastes they promise. My favorite honey is the light, delicately flavored thyme honey; Harold's the robust, winey capping honey. To pour over my griddle cakes, we both agree, there could be no better choice than syrupy buckwheat honey. (Honeys take their names from the plants from which the bees select their pollen.)

Add one more attribute of honey: it attracts water, and helps keep breads and cakes moist and fresh.

And add a caution: buy only uncooked, unfiltered honey. Cooking destroys flavor and nutrients, and filtering removes the health-packed pollen particles. Uncooked, unfiltered honey is available mainly in health-food stores. The highly processed supermarket honeys we've tasted are cloyingly sweet, textured like ointment, and sometimes unpleasantly medicinal in taste. If that's the only kind of honey you've ever tasted, you're ready to discover a whole new world of sweetness. Use honey, as I do, in limited quantities.

About sugar substitutes. Non-caloric sweeteners, like saccharin and cyclamates, although not strong carcinogens, do pose a potential risk for cancer to some individuals, according to reports from the National Cancer Institute and the Food and Drug Administration. Two eight-ounce diet soft drinks a day could increase the risk of developing bladder cancer by 60%. Caloric diet sweeteners—xylitol, mannitol, and sorbitol—have a tendency to induce diarrhea. For my comments on fructose, see page 228. No sugar substitute ranks higher than 0 on my taste meter.

What About Fiber?

Fiber can be regarded as a non-caloric complex carbohydrate. It is the indigestible residue of plants—what grandma used to call "roughage." Long regarded as a non-nutrient, it is now known to play a significant role in the body's biochemistry.

There's a plentiful supply of fiber in Diet for Life menus—in whole-grain cereals, breads, seeds, fruits, vegetables, and nuts—and we see no need for supplements. (Fiber pills have no verified nutritional or medical properties.)

Here's a rundown on the kinds of fiber, the foods containing them, and what science has discovered about the effects of different kinds of fiber on your health.

The water-soluble fibers. These are pectins (the same substances used to make jellies) and gums. These fibers are reported to lower blood cholesterol and triglycerides, and help control blood-sugar levels in diabetics. (Bran has none of these therapeutic effects.) Good sources of pectins are apples, bananas, cabbage, carrots, grapes, and oranges; of gums, beans, oatmeal, and sesame seeds.

The water-insoluble fibers. These are cellulose (the same substance of which wood is mainly composed), hemi-cellulose, and lignin. They are excellent means of countering constipation. Bran, which is mostly cellulose, is the best of all natural laxatives (it softens the stool and makes it easier to pass). Fresh carrots, cabbage, and apples (be sure to eat the skin) are runners-up. Insoluble fibers are effective aids to elimination only when they're coarse. Applesauce, for example, is a less effective laxative than a whole apple. Perversely, finely ground bran can cause constipation.

Good sources of cellulose are apples (unpeeled), bran (coarse), carrots (fresh), and pears (unpeeled); of hemi-cellulose, bran (cereals), eggplant, radishes, and whole-grain breads; of lignin, pears, potatoes (browned), and whole-grain breads (toasted).

All fibers can absorb large amounts of water, so they give a feeling of fullness, which is of particular value on a calorie-restricted diet.

There is some evidence (though it's disputed) that high-fiber diets can be helpful in the treatment of spastic colon, and other intestinal diseases, including regional enteritis (Chrohn's disease), and diverticulitis, which painfully affects many people of middle age. But there is no evidence to back up claims that such diets can effectively treat appendicitis, hemorrhoids, varicose veins, cancer of the colon, and heart attack.

Prolonged consumption of excess fiber can be harmful. Intestinal bacteria attacks fiber, sometimes producing gas, with consequent pain, vomiting, and nausea. Absorption of essential minerals by the body can be impaired, as well.

Certainly, fiber has been neglected in the American diet. In the Diet for Life its rightful place has been restored. But fiber, although it has some health-promoting qualities, is no cure-all.

11

The Magic of Herbs and Spices

People all over the world throughout the ages have regarded herbs and spices as magic. I can testify that they are in the kitchen. And there's a growing body of evidence to support the health-promoting qualities of some herbs and spices—qualities which appeared magical in the pre-scientific world. Of all herbs and spices, there's none more magical medicinally and gastronomically than—

Garlic: The Wonder Herb

Dr. Hans Reuter of Cologne, Germany, in 1978, announced the results of a series of clinical investigations that proved garlic can clear blood vessels of fat, and markedly lower blood cholesterol. He reported, as well, that garlic can kill off bacteria, including those causing diphtheria and tuberculosis, more effectively in some cases than penicillin and other conventional antibiotics. One antibiotic so widely used in the Soviet Union that it's called "Russian penicillin" is allicin, an extract of garlic.

In 1980, the Hunan Medical College in Changsha, China, documented overwhelming success in treating with garlic alone a frequently fatal form of meningitis, a fungus-induced inflammation of the brain and spinal cord. The disease had been treated previously with a costly anti-fungicide which reduced fatalities by only 15%, and produced such side effects as convulsions, kidney malfunctions, and generalized pain.

There is medical evidence to indicate, as well, that garlic can be helpful or effective in the treatment of intestinal infections by parasites; atherosclerosis, coronary thrombosis, and high blood pressure; anemia, arthritis, abnormal blood-pressure levels, and other ailments.

Garlic's therapeutic properties have been known to folklore medicine for thousands of years, and immortalized in the legend of the vampire, who is repelled by the sight of garlic. The vampire in Latin is *nosferatu,* which means "the bringer of disease"; and garlic is the magic charm that keeps disease away.

It also keeps everybody away when it's not used properly. A retired philosophy professor, who eats oodles of raw garlic because he believes it keeps him healthy, recently was barred from riding on Long Island buses because his breath was more foul than even the exhaust fumes of the buses. I use a great deal of garlic, but it's never detectable on our breath. For alliumphiles (garlic lovers) who sneak through life with a pocketful of Clorets and a guilty expression, here's the secret:

Throw away your garlic press. Instead, *mince* the bulbs. (Mincing means cutting into pieces less than ⅛" on a side.) Use in conjunction with parsley; it's a natural odor killer. And never, never, never eat garlic raw. Garlic-free breath is that simple.

Garlic is my first response to: "What do you do when you don't use salt?" This lusciously pungent herb spikes up many of my dishes, and it gives them the tang (although not the taste) of salt. Yet, you'll never taste garlic as such. Each of my recipes is choreographed to produce a single grand extravaganza; and no one ingredient—especially garlic—ever showboats on its own to spoil the ensemble.

Garlic is a member of the lily family. So are onions, shallots, chives, and leeks, all of which are reported to have medicinal properties similar to garlic's, albeit of lesser magnitude; and all of which to some degree echo garlic's brazen pizzazz. Like garlic, you'll find them in the cast of a long string of my successes; and, like garlic, they should be minced, and meshed with other ingredients, to subordinate their self-expression.

The Gourmet Health-Conscious Shopper's Guide to Herbs and Spices

I use a bevy of herbs and spices. They do much more than just compensate for saltlessness. They extend the range of human taste experience almost to infinity. They're sweet and they're pungent; they're delicate and they're rough; they're exotic and they're familiar; they're docile and they're assertive; they're piquant and they're mellow; they're elegant and they're down to earth; they're fragrant, titillating, colorful, aromatic—they're everything a food lover can dream of, and more. Their combinations are seemingly endless. Mixing them into potpourris of goodness, and matching those blendings to the bounty of land and sea, is, to the dedicated cook, one of the most sublime of all challenges.

An herb is a barkless seed plant, characterized by a special scent or flavor. A spice is an aromatic seed, nut, leaf, or vegetable, usually ground.

If folklore is to be believed, herbs and spices comprise a *materia medica* of marvelous cures for all the ailments known to man. Beneath this monumental exaggeration, there's a solid bedrock on which to build a case for the health-promotion qualities of these taste-tinglers. In refrigerator-less times, spices preserved foods against the onslaughts of fungi and bacteria. Some spice oils are powerful germicides. Vitamin-potent (paprika is one of the most concentrated sources of vitamin C), spices are devoid of calories, and virtually free of sodium.

As rich in vitamins, richer in minerals, and almost as sparing in sodium and calories as spices, herbs are pharmacological factories from which scientists have extracted many valuable drugs: ephedrine (for the relief of nasal congestion); digitalis (a heart stimulant); quinine (an anti-malarial); and rauwolfia (a blood-pressure depressant), to name only a few. The very word "drug" comes from the old Anglo-Saxon for "dry"—and "dry" referred to dried herbs which were used as "simples" (remedies).

In the kitchen, fresh herbs, by and large, are preferable to dried herbs; and if you can grow them, or buy them, do so. Many of us can't. Then dried herbs are perfectly satisfactory. Vitamins are lost or depleted, but minerals are concentrated, and medicinal properties are purported to be enhanced. Flavors shade off into unexpected and delightful nuances; and many truly sophisticated herb lovers deliberately choose the dried variant over the fresh herb. The long shelf life of dried herbs (about six months) is in their favor, too.

Now meet the herbs and spices used most frequently in the Diet for Life. Their medical characteristics which I've listed have been culled from herbal lore not scientific journals, and must be assessed on that basis. *Arrangement is alphabetical, and an asterisk (*) after a name distinguishes a spice from an herb.*

Allspice* is sweet and pungent, combining the flavors of cinnamon, nutmeg, and cloves (hence, its name). But it's a single spice, not a mixture. It's a tonic to the digestive system. It adds zest to my pastries, desserts, and marinades.

Anise seeds* have a pleasant, warm licorice flavor. They aid digestion, stimulate the appetite, and sweeten the breath. I use it in breads, cakes, and desserts; and in my fish dishes.

Basil, or Sweet Basil, is, as its alternate name proclaims, sweet. But it's also spicy and clove-like, and exudes an alluring perfume which the whole Italian nation adores, and so do we. It's a tonic, a stimulant, and a digestive; and it fights bad breath. It enlivens my marinades, omelettes, and sauces, especially those for pasta; and it marries heavenly with tomatoes, raw or cooked, in a paste or a purée.

Bay leaves are moderately sweet with a hint of astringency, and an ever so slight bitter undertaste. They improve the digestion and stimulate the appetite. They perform wonders in the preparation of fish.

*Caraway seeds** are sharp and pungent, and give Jewish and Norwegian rye breads their distinctive flavor. They're a tonic for the organs of digestion. (The reason they're in those breads?) My light, airy ryes don't need digestive aids, but I add caraway seeds to tickle the tongue. I also use them in dips.

*Cardamom seeds** are as hot as ginger. They're an anti-acid. I use them to add a tantalizing touch of the Punjab to breads; and they haunt the heart of my Indian dishes.

*Cayenne (red pepper)** is sweet as an angel at first bite, but devilishly pepperish thereafter. It has antiseptic properties and a salutory effect on the circulatory system. It adds the bite of a pitchfork to some of my sauces, marinades, and dips.

*Chili con carne seasoning** is a fiery mixture of cumin, garlic, coriander, oregano, and ground dried chili pods. (Don't confuse it with chili con carne *powder,* which contains salt and black pepper, both nutritional castoffs from the Diet for Life.) The chili comes from a large group of peppers, the capsicums, which produce spices which vary from mild paprika to the hot chilis of Latin America. Some of the more torrid capsicum spices have found their way into this chili seasoning. Chili is regarded as a stimulant; and additional health-promoting properties are contributed by this seasoning's other ingredients. Chili con carne seasoning provides a touch of the tropics in my sauces and marinades.

Chives taste like onions grown for the Upper East Side crowd. Its antiseptic and appetite-stimulating powers head a long list of medicinal attributes. It adds a light onion flavor to the blandest of vegetables (it's an exquisite complement to a simple baked potato), and it's an applause-getter in omelettes and dips.

*Cinnamon** is sweet, highly aromatic, and somewhat astringent. It's a balm for the stomach, and relieves gas. It works wonders with breakfast cereals, puddings, pies, desserts, and low-fat milk drinks.

*Cloves** give that special strong flavor and aroma to roast ham. It has a reputation of being an enemy of aches and pains. I use it to wake up almost any kind of dish.

*Coriander seeds** are bitter-sweet, with a fresh, delicate spring-like aroma. They're an aid to the digestion, and are purported to strengthen the heart. The toasted seeds are flavor-enhanced; and that's how I use them in my breads.

*Cumin** is sharp and astringent, but pleasantly so. It has food preservative properties, and is probably bactericidal. It adds the flavor of faraway places to my Indian-style dishes.

Curry powder*, no salt or pepper added, is a fiery blend of cardamom, coriander, cumin, dill, fenugreek, and turmeric. It tastes and looks like . . . well, curry. For the medicinal properties of the other spices, see under their individual listings; but don't look for fenugreek. I don't like the odor or the taste, so it's not listed. The chemical composition of the seeds is close to that of cod-liver oil. Fenugreek is a general tonic, promoting the health, in particular, of the stomach, intestines, and nerves.

Dill tastes like a pickling spice (and the seeds are just that). It is a carminative (a substance which helps expel stomach gas); and it improves the health of nerves, nails, and hair. I use the leaves in salads, and as a garnish for all types of entrées and side dishes. I use little dried dill because its sodium content is on the high side; and I don't often use dill seeds because, except in a pickling broth, they're shy of flavor.

Fennel seeds*, like anise seeds, have a warm, sweet taste reminiscent of licorice. They aid in the digestion of cabbage, peas, beans, cheese, and especially oily fish. It makes sense to include fennel seeds in my recipes for those potential digestion-disturbers, and I do, with an exciting flavor bonus as a reward.

Garlic is *the* indispensable herb. You've read about its multifarious virtues earlier in this chapter.

Ginger* is hot and pungent, with an underlying impish sweetness. It's a stimulating, warming digestive, and can act as a mild laxative. It puts a kick into all sorts of recipes of mine, from cakes to marinades.

Juniper berries* have a warm, pungent taste—the dominant flavoring of gin. They're a diuretic and a stimulant. I use them in several sophisticated chicken dishes.

Mace.* See *Nutmeg.*

Marjoram is delicately sweet and minty. It is prescribed for sour stomach, bad breath, and other digestive ailments. It's just right for lamb and poultry, and brings a surprise taste thrill to my innovative rice dishes.

Mint is cool, sharp, and clean on the tongue. There are two kinds of mint: peppermint, and spearmint. Both are breath-fresheners, fight stomach gases and acid stomach, and in general have a beneficial effect on the digestive system. I use peppermint, the more robust-flavored of the two mints, as a soothing tea; as a garnish for meats, particularly lamb; and to impart a minty nuance to my sauces and marinades.

Mustard seeds* are stingingly hot. They increase the appetite, fight flatulence (gas in the stomach) and halitosis (bad breath), and have some antiseptic value. The seeds, which are black and white, are ground to a powder and mixed with a variety of other spices, vinegar, and/or wine to produce prepared mustards. Harold enjoys a salt-free Dijon mustard to perk up leftovers (it's obtainable from gourmet shops). In my marinades and sauces, mustard powder (not prepared mustard) is mingled subtly with other ingredients, and never dominates.

*Nutmeg** is exotically sweet and pungent. Mace, which is made from the dried shell of the nutmeg, is slightly stronger. Both spices have antiseptic properties. Both are valuable offbeat sweeteners for my cakes, pies, sauces, and marinades.

Onion, although usually regarded as a vegetable, is the coarsest member of the herbaceous garlic family, as its eye-stinging qualities readily attest to. It's an antiseptic, helps control blood pressure, and fights thrombosis (blood-clotting in the circulatory system, which can lead to heart attack). Cooked, it sweetens; and the sweet and acrid oniony flavor adds savor to omelettes, stews, sauces, marinades, and to many of my super-tasty breads and rolls.

Oregano, the pizza herb, is wild marjoram, and, like all feral things, is far more macho than its civilized counterpart. For medical uses, oregano has it all over marjoram, adding to the more delicate herb's list of credits: effectiveness in fighting headaches, toothaches, and the aches of rheumatism. Fresh oregano is rare in Manhattan; and dried oregano is a disappointingly weak-flavored herb. But the dried variety, blended with other herbs and spices, helps me recapture the gusto of the cooking of southern Italy; and that's the way I use it.

*Paprika** is the mildest of all spices made from the capsicums (see *Chili con carne seasoning*), but it's still sharp. It's an excellent digestive, producing a pleasant feeling of warmth in the stomach and a general glow of well-being. I use it to give the gypsy flavor to chicken and a wide variety of other dishes.

Parsley is a mellow, clean-tasting green. It comes in two varieties: *curly,* which makes an attractive garnish, and *flat* which is more aromatic, and easier to mince. It's a remedy for digestive ailments, bladder and kidney complaints, and helps keep the breath fresh. When added to dishes featuring members of the garlic family, it blends well, and overcomes residual mouth odors. There are virtually none of my recipes, except for sweets and baked goods, which do not call for parsley as an ingredient or as a garnish; and my green sauces are built around it. Don't simply enjoy parsley as a garnish—eat it! Its gentle freshness heightens the flavor of the dish.

*Pickling spices** are combined commercially. The mix consists of allspice, bay leaves, cayenne pepper, cloves, coriander, dill, ginger, mustard seeds—all of which are listed alphabetically in this chapter—

as well as cassia, fenugreek, and black pepper. Cassia, Chinese cinnamon, is a harsh-flavored cinnamon. Fenugreek, intensely and distinctively aromatic, is described under *Curry powder*. Black pepper is acceptable here because the quantity is minute; otherwise, it's banned from the Diet for Life because some experts feel that in some cases it may heighten blood pressure.

Poppy seeds* have a perfumed fruity flavor. They're considered a tonic food, with the special quality of soothing raw nerves. They're used in my cuisine to add an eye- and tongue-pleasing garnish to cakes and breads.

Rosemary is a hearty, fragrant relative of the mints. It has just a shade of bitterness. Like garlic, it has a reputation as a cure-all (but, unlike garlic, the reputation is not supported by scientific studies; at least, not yet). Rosemary is best known pharmaceutically as a treatment for heart ailments and female complaints, and as an antidote to fatigue and forgetfulness. Rosemary adds special luster to our chicken dishes, and it sparkles in my marinades.

Sage, the Thanksgiving turkey herb, is related to the mints. Like rosemary, another minty herb, it has been regarded for centuries as a panacea, remedying everything from snake bite to the decay of old age. Not the least of its purported virtues is its ability to spark the intellect, which may be why it's called sage. I use sage in my recipes for turkey—it's a sage tradition—and for other poultry, as well.

Savory, sweet and tangy, is a minty herb. It tones the digestive system and fights flatulence. So it's fortunate it marries so well gustatorially with beans. It also reduces the tell-tale cooking odors of cabbage, Brussels sprouts, and turnips.

Shallots, small-bulbed and delicate, are the most subtley-flavored of all members of the garlic clan. Medicinal properties are onion-like, but to a markedly lesser degree. Use shallots and garlic in tandem, my style, and you'll never crave salt again.

Tarragon is sweet and licorice-like with a mild bite. It's one of those wonder herbs that is supposed to cure everything. Increasing stamina is its feature attribute. It's anise-like flavor makes it just right for some of my fish dishes, and its spicy sweetness gives added life to some of my cooked vegetables.

Thyme is the clam chowder herb. Because it's so marvelously aromatic and sweet, it has become the base for many liqueurs, including Benedictine. It's supposed to help almost all digestive complaints, and set right many nervous-type ailments, including nervous indigestion, nightmares, and sick headaches. Walk in when I'm making my stews, and fish and fowl dishes, and you'll catch me with thyme on my hands!

Watercress has a biting, tangy taste, and a pleasant flesh-like texture. It's a blood tonic and an anemia remedy; it strengthens the heart and the eyes; and it combats nervous disorders. Rich in vitamins, minerals, and proteins, this basically complex-carbohydrate food is, to some herbalists, the best salad green known to man. It may also very well be the best tasting. Its brilliant green leaves make a lovely garnish; and by itself or in harmony with sparklingly fresh tomatoes, it cooks into unforgettable soups.

REPEAT: The herbal remedies in the foregoing list are not represented as bona fide cures or as substitutes for reputable medical therapies. They're presented as medical folklore curiosa. But, based solely on our experience, it would seem that the judicious use of herbs and spices in the kitchen could have a salutary effect on the digestive system. During the time of his heart attack, and for months thereafter, Harold was beset with stomach disorders and frequent intense and incapacitating eruptions of flatulence (probably related to an atherosclerotic condition, his cardiologist surmised). But those maladies are only memories now.

But whether herbs and spices have specific pharmacological properties or not, they do make healthful food taste better. And how can that not make you feel good? And how can feeling good be bad for you?

12

Fat-Containing Foods You Can Live With

An optimum amount of fat—about 20% of the total caloric intake on the Diet for Life—is required to keep your body operating at peak efficiency. But if you're an average American, you'll find it next to impossible to hold your fat intake down that low, unless you—

Beware of Hidden Fats

Just as there is hidden salt and sugar in virtually every commercial-food product, so is there hidden fat, and usually of the wrong kind. You'll find hidden fat even where you least expect it—in health-food restaurant dishes. Here's a sampling from typical menus (fat calories are expressed in percentage of total calories contributed by the food):

1. *Avocado* is about 75% fat, about ⅔ of which is saturated.
2. *Broiled fish* is about 50% fat. The butter or margarine with which it is cooked make up the major fat contribution.
3. *Granola* (commercial) is about 33% fat, which comes from added oil, and the fats in nuts, seeds, and coconut (one of the most saturated-fat-rich foods found in nature). By comparison, most of the commercial breakfast cereals shunned by health-food addicts contain virtually no fat. (They do contain sugar, but so do most commercial granolas, although under an alias. Turbinado sugar *is* sugar.)
4. *Quiche* is made with cheese, cream, and pie crust. The cheese is about 75% fat, the cream 100% fat, and the pie crust about 50% fat.

5. *Salad dressings*—tofu herb, tahini, or Italian vinaigrette—are about 80% fat.

6. *Tahini custard* is about 83% fat.

7. *Vegetarian vegetable soup* is about 35% fat, due mostly to added oils.

8. *Yogurt* is about 50% fat, and most of the fat is saturated.

Other health-food restaurant menu items loaded with fat are: vegetable soy burgers topped with melted cheese (the soy is the fattest of all beans); rice with tahini béchamel (with as much fat as the real béchamel); crêpes (made with fatty egg yolks); and "natural" cakes (which contain highly saturated coconut and palm oils).

Health-food restaurant dishes also contain high amounts of hidden salt, and not inconsiderable amounts of hidden sugar. The sophisticated health-conscious gourmet is likely to find the food in health-food restaurants as unhealthful as it is unpalatable.

But no matter where you eat, including your home, if you're not on the Diet for Life or another low-fat diet, 45% of your daily caloric intake is derived from fat, the bulk of which is hidden. A far lower fat intake is necessary to help ward off degenerative diseases, and to maintain your weight, your health, and your vitality.

You also need the right kind of fats.

There are *three kinds* distinguished by their chemical makeup. All three kinds have pairs of slots which can be filled with hydrogen. When all pairs are filled (that is to say, when the fat is saturated with hydrogen), the fat is called *saturated.* (Hydrogenated fats are those to which hydrogen has been added artificially to fill all or most of the slots.) When only one pair is unfilled, the fat is called *monounsaturated.* When more than one pair is unfilled, the fat is called *polyunsaturated;* and the more unfilled pairs, the more polyunsaturated the fat.

In general, saturated fats are bad for you, polyunsaturated fats are good for you, and monounsaturated fats are neutral. Most fat-containing foods are mixtures of the three kinds of fats. What the health-conscious food lover looks for is the ratio of polyunsaturated fat to saturated fat; the higher the ratio, the more polyunsaturated fat the food contains, and the better the food is for you.

Here are the fat-containing foods which contribute the right amounts of fats; and the amounts of the two active kinds of fats which, averaged out over a week's Diet for Life menus, provide a satisfactorily high ratio of polyunsaturated fat to saturated fat. They're the kinds of foods to which you have become accustomed: meats, fish, poultry, dairy products, and oils. There are no kooky foods in the Diet for Life.

As you become acquainted with the truth about fat-containing foods, you'll find, as we did, many surprises. You should know, for example, that some fish are fatty, that Jarlsberg is not a low-fat cheese, and that—

Lean Meat Can Be Healthful

There is nothing wrong with meat as such, as long as it is part of a balanced diet. We're carnivores by nature; and the human race has survived for 12,000,000 years or so subsisting for the most part on meat. What *is* wrong is the way we grow our livestock. Feedstuffs and hormone injections are bio-engineered to produce unnaturally obese animals. The marbling of our meat is a gross abnormality— and a dangerous one. Not only does the normal prime cut contribute about 75% of its total calories in fat, but most of those calories are derived from saturated fat.

Naturally lean meat, on the other hand, is a superb food, high in protein and essential vitamins and minerals. Members of some African tribes, who sustain themselves in large part on grass-fed cattle, live healthy, long lives, utterly untouched by heart attack or other degenerative diseases. That kind of meat is impossible to obtain in the supermarket. But lean cuts are available; and some, when properly cooked, have less fat than an equivalent amount of fish broiled with butter.

The Gourmet Fat-Conscious Shopper's Guide to the Meat Market

In this guide, as in all other guides in this chapter, the food is classified according to fat content in four categories. The fat content is expressed as percentage of total calories. The categories are:

- *Very low fat:* 0 to 11%
- *Low fat:* 11 to 30%
- *Lean:* 31 to 40%
- *Medium fat:* 41 to 49%

Edibles with fat content above 50% do not appear in my guides, and are to be shunned as regular fare. The fat contents in the following *Guide to the Meat Market* have been calculated for choice cuts of raw beef and lamb, and equivalent grades of raw veal, pork, venison, and rabbit.

BEEF

If you've been told to restrict your meat dishes to veal, here's an eye-opener: two choice cuts of beef, round and hindshank, are lower in fat than veal. They're even lower in fat than low-fat yogurt and tofu.

- *Very low fat:*   None
- *Low fat:*   None
- *Lean:*   Roast beef (round) and London broil (hindshank), 31%. Pot roast (foreshank), 33%. Flank steak and sirloin steak (wedge or round bone), 36%. Hamburger ground from any of the foregoing cuts. But beware of pre-ground "lean" hamburger; it contains 50% fat or more.
- *Medium fat:*   Chuck and double-bone sirloin, 42%; Rump, 43%; Porterhouse (which includes filet mignon, shell steak, and tail steak), 45%; T-bone steak and short plate, 45%.

VEAL

Veal is not, as many dieter's believe, a synonym for lean meat. A calf is a Jack Sprat animal—it's lean and fat, and nothing in between. And when it's fat, it's very, very fat. Breast of veal is 70% fat; and the flank, which is lean in the full-grown cow, is 50% fat.

- *Very low fat:*   None
- *Low fat:*   None
- *Lean:*   Leg (foreshank), 35%; Shoulder chops and chuck, 39%; Loin chops and other loin cuts, 40%; Round and rump, 40%
- *Medium fat:*   None

LAMB

Lamb chops have long been a standby of high-protein diets. But only one cut of chops qualified as lean meat.

- *Very low fat:*   None
- *Low fat:*   None
- *Lean:*   Leg, 36%; Loin chops and other loin cuts, 40%
- *Medium fat:*   Shoulder chops, 47%; Rib chops, 48%

PORK

Pork, as you've known all along, is a fatty meat. But two types of pork fall into our *Lean* category; and that's fortunate, because this is a delicious meat, and as rich a source of B vitamins as you can find. Pork chops as a class do not ordinarily qualify for any of our four acceptable categories, but some individual chops do. Make the eye test when shopping. If the chops don't look fatty, chances are they're not. We've bought pork chops that don't ooze any fat at all when they are broiled.

- *Very low fat:* None
- *Low fat:* None
- *Lean:* Picnic pork, 37%; Fresh ham, 40%
- *Medium fat:* None

VENISON and RABBIT

If these meats are among your favorites, here's good news. The fat content of venison is a little under 30%, and of rabbit, a little over. They're the leanest of meats.

FAT-WISE HINTS ABOUT MEATS

- Use your eyes when you shop. Avoid marbled meats. Select meats that don't look fatty.
- Tenderize *Lean* meat by marinating, braising, or pounding (as for veal scallopine). Don't use tenderizers.
- Before cooking, trim off excess fat.
- Decrease the fat content of meats by broiling or grilling (fat drips off); or by braising, then chilling, and removing the fat layer that forms on top.
- Eat meat only twice a week (it's best as a dinner entrée), and never on consecutive days. We've established these limitations not only because of the amount of fat, but because the fat is mostly saturated. In even the leanest beef or veal cuts, there's only a trace of polyunsaturated fat. In the leanest of pork cuts, the ratio of saturated fat to polyunsaturated fat is 3:1; and it's 10:1 in the leanest cuts of lamb. We never eat meat on consecutive days because we're wary of the cumulative effects of saturated fats.
- Eat more *Lean* meat than *Medium fat.*

Fish Can Be Fat

Many health-food devotees live with two myths about fish: 1. all fish is lean; 2. all fish is highly polyunsaturated. Here's why they're myths.

All fish is not lean. In terms of percentage of total calories, shad, sardines, lake whitefish, and smelts are 50% fat; Greenland halibut, 51%; rainbow or steelhead trout, 53%; lake trout, 54%; dogfish, 55%; Atlantic mackerel, 59%; Atlantic herring, 60%; Chinook (King) salmon, 63%; spot, 65%; sablefish, 71%; and gizzard shad, a whopping 83%.

But the majority of piscatorial species available in the U.S.A. contain no more than 30% fat; and many contain less than 10%.

Fish is not high in polyunsaturated fats. On the average, only 44% of fish fat is polyunsaturated. Safflower oil, by comparison, is 78% polyunsaturated.

But of the high-protein foods—meat, fish, and poultry—fish is overall the highest in polyunsaturated fats, and the lowest in total fat.

The Gourmet Fat-Conscious Shopper's Guide to the Fish Market

In this guide, fish are arranged alphabetically within the four categories. A separate guide for *Shellfish, Etc.*, follows the fourth category.

GUIDE FOR FISH

- *Very low fat:* Abalone, 5%; Burbot, 10%; Cod, 4%; Flounder, 9%; Gray snapper, 9%; Haddock, 1%; Hake, 3%; Perch (yellow), 9%; Pike, 9%; Pollock, 9%; Red snapper, 9%; Sea bass (white), 5%; Scrod, 4%; Skate, 7%; Sole, 9%; Soursop, 4%; Tile fish, 7%

- *Low fat:* Albacore, 12%; Barracuda (Pacific), 21%; Bass (sea), 12%; Bass (small-mouth or large-mouth), 22%; Bass (striped), 23%; Bass (white), 21%; Bluefish, 25%; Carp, 26%; Catfish (freshwater), 27%; Croaker (Atlantic), 20%; Halibut, 11%; Herring (Pacific), 24%; Redfish (ocean perch), 12%; Perch (white), 30%; Porgy, 27%; Rockfish, 17%; Salmon, pink, 27%; Scup, 27%; Smelt, 20%; Sturgeon, 20%; Trout (brook), 19%; Tuna (bluefin), 25%; Tuna (yellowfin), 20%; Wreckfish, 20%; Whiting, 20%

- *Lean:* Alewife, 35%; Buffalofish, 33%; Swordfish, 31%; Yellowtail (Pacific), 35%

- *Medium fat:* Butterfish, 43%; Mackerel (Pacific), 41%; Mullet, 43%; Salmon (Atlantic), 45%; Weakfish, 42%

SHELLFISH, ETC.

ETC. means: frogs' legs, snails, octopus, and squid. They're included here because, like shellfish, they're non-scaled, non-finned, non-gilled food items sold in the fish market. One ETC. not listed is eel because of its high fat content, 70%.

GUIDE TO SHELLFISH

- *Very low fat:* Crab, 11%; Crayfish, 6%; Frogs' legs, 4%; Lobster (spiny), 6%; Octopus, 10%; Shrimp, 8%; Snails, 14%; Squid, 10%.

- *Low fat:* Clams, 21%; Lobster, 20%; Mussels, 21%; Oysters (Eastern), 25%; Oysters (Pacific and Western), 22%

- *Lean:* None
- *Medium fat* None

FAT-WISE HINTS ABOUT FISH

- Don't eat the skin; it's fatty.
- Trim away excess fat before cooking.
- Don't cook with butter or too much margarine or oil. It makes little sense to buy a fish for its low-fat content, then add excessive amounts of fat.
- Concentrate on fish in the *Very low fat* category. They're as inexpensive as they are delicious. One of our favorites is tile fish. It feeds on the crustacea at the bottom of the sea, and tastes like them. (See my recipe on page 98.)

You Can Enjoy Poultry

Don't let chicken fat turn you away from eating poultry. The light meat of some chickens falls into the *Low fat* category. Cornish hens, which are young, tiny chickens, are even leaner. And the white meat of a young turkey contains only 3% fat, less than any fish, except hake (1%). But there are several fat fowl, capon (70% fat), duck (79% fat), and goose (85% fat). None appears on the following list of poultry acceptables. (Duck is also phenomenally high in cholesterol.) Of the birds on our list, chicken, rock Cornish hen, and turkey are our favorites.

The Gourmet Fat-Conscious Shopper's Guide to the Poultry Market

GUIDE TO POULTRY

- *Very low fat:* Turkey (young; 24 weeks old or younger), light meat, 3%; Turkey (26-32 weeks), light meat, 8%; Cornish hen, probably 6%
- *Low fat:* Chicken (fryer), light meat, 13%; Chicken (roaster), light meat, 23%; Turkey (young; 24 weeks or younger), dark meat, 20%; Turkey (26-32 weeks), dark meat, 30%
- *Lean:* Chicken (fryer), dark meat, 31%; Chicken (roaster), dark meat, 32%; Quail, 36%; Pheasant, 40%
- *Medium fat:* Squab, 48%

FAT-WISE HINTS ABOUT POULTRY

- When shopping for chickens, remember fryers are less fatty than roasters. But don't fry them.
- When shopping for turkey, remember young birds are less fatty than older birds.
- Remove the skin from chickens and Cornish hens before cooking. It can reduce fat by as much as 25% of the total weight of the bird.

- Melt off fat in a broiler; or skim off fat that rises to the top after stewing and refrigerating.
- It's not possible to make a decent-tasting turkey with skin removed prior to cooking. Instead, puncture (with a skewer) the skin first and then roast. A good deal of the fat will drip off.

The Truth About Low-Fat Cheese

Jarlsberg is a part-skim-milk cheese. It has a fat content *(matière grasse)* of 5%.

Brie is a *double crème* (double fat) cheese. It has a fat content *(matière grasse)* of 75%.

Which is the fattier cheese?

Let's find out the *true* fat content of each cheese. The fat content as given refers to the percentage of fat in the solid, or dry, matter of the cheese. (The cheese industry's designation for fat content is %IDM—percent in dry matter.) Water is the other component of a cheese. The more dry matter in a cheese, the more fat it will contain by weight.

In every 100 grams of Jarlsberg, there are 50 grams of dry matter. Fat is 56% of the dry matter, so the number of grams of fat in 100 grams of Jarlsberg is 28 (56% of 50). That's the same as saying the cheese is 28% fat by weight (28 divided by 100).

In every 100 grams of Brie, there are 33 grams of dry matter. Fat is 75% of the dry matter, so the number of grams of fat in 100 grams of Brie is about 25 (75% of 33). That's the same as saying the cheese is about 25% fat by weight (about 25 divided by 100).

Final results:

Brie: 25% fat by weight. Jarlsberg: 28%.

Jarlsberg is fattier.

Jarlsberg has about the same fat content by weight as many other cheeses generally regarded as fatty as Brie, including Gruyère, Muenster, Gorgonzola, Cheddar, and processed American cheese.

Why is Jarlsberg, then, called part-skim? Because the designation of a cheese is derived from the kind of milk product with which the manufacturing process *begins:* in this case, part-skim milk. But whole milk and cream are added *during* the process to bring fat content up to industry standards, and where applicable, government standards for fat content. Most part-skim- or skim-milk cheeses are as fatty as whole-milk cheeses.

The point is: you can't tell from industry terms used to describe a cheese and define its fat content whether a cheese is low-fat.

What about cheeses labeled "low-fat"? They're processed cheeses. Some are made here; some come from abroad. The fat content of the American variety is about ⅓ less than that of regular cheese. But you can eat American low-fat cheese only if you have a passion for semi-congealed mucilage. In the European variety, fat is not reduced; cholesterol is. In the processing, some of the butterfat, which is high in cholesterol, is replaced by vegetable fat with a cholesterol content of nil. Cheeses like Swiss Lorraine and Swiss Chris, which are advertised as low-fat, are in reality low-cholesterol cheeses.

Aren't there any palatable true low-fat cheeses? We wish there were more than there are. Aside from its high amount of saturated fat (15 to 20 times its polyunsaturated fat content), cheese is an admirable food. It is rich in protein, contains all the fat-soluble vitamins (A, D, E, and K) and the fat to dissolve them, and has three times the amount of B-complex vitamins found in milk. It feeds into the bloodstream slowly, staving off hunger signals (which is why its been a perennial on high-protein/high-fat reducing diets). And the varieties of cheese to delight the tongue are almost as extensive as the varieties of wine, with which they form a perfect blendship.

Here is a list of the few true low-fat cheeses available in this country. You'll have to hunt down most of them in gourmet and cheese shops; and whether you think it's worth the trouble will depend upon your taste buds. There are some we can't stomach (Harzer Händkäse, for one), and some we can't do without (Sap Sago is superb on my pasta sauces). We eat *Very low fat* cheeses routinely; and we nibble on others, as-is or gussied up, mainly as hors d'oeuvres. Gjetost is a superb dessert cheese; but it's in the high-medium-fat range, so use small quantities only.

The Gourmet Fat-Conscious Shopper's Guide to Low-Fat Cheese

There isn't sufficient information available to calculate fat content as percentage of total calories for individual cheeses. But as a rule of thumb, cheeses between 15-20% IDM fall into the *Medium fat (high)* category; between 5-15%, in the *Medium fat (low)* category; and below 5% in the *Low fat* category.

In that latter category, two cheeses stand out for their sparseness of fat. One is the familiar dry-curd cottage cheese, in which fat contributes only 3% of the total calories. The other is the unfamiliar Sap Sago, a clover-flavored Swiss cheese so hard it can only be used when grated; this contains no fat at all.

Regular domestic and imported cheeses, including many part-skims and skims, have IDM's over 20%, and percentage of fat calories ranging from 60% to 74%. They are, of course, excluded from our guide. But if you're a cheese lover, take mini-nibbles of your favorites once a day when you're on your maintenance diet. The operative phrases in the preceding sentence are: *maintenance diet; mini-nibbles; once a day.*

GUIDE TO CHEESES

- *Very low fat:* Cottage cheese, dry curd, less than ½% milkfat; Farmer cheese; Gammelöst; Pot cheese; Sap Sago
- *Low fat:* None
- *Lean:* None
- *Medium fat:* Appenzeller Räss; Harzer Händkäse; St. Otho
  (low)
- *Medium fat:* Gjetost; Livarot; Maigrichon; Magriotte; Monvelay Al-
  (high) légé; Part-skim Mozzarella (the low-moisture variety is somewhat higher in fat); Parmesan; Reggiano; Romano

All About Yogurt, Non-Fat Milk, and Buttermilk

Yogurt. Add bacteria—*Lactobacillus bulgaricus* or *Streptococcus thermophilus*—to skim, low-fat, or whole milk, and you get a thick, custardy food with an acrid, metallic taste. That's yogurt. Elie Metchnikoff, a noted Russian biologist, thought it was the secret of eternal life. He lived on it, and died at the age of 71. Yogurt is purported to be the perfect food, and the dieter's best friend. It is said to lower cholesterol levels, fight heart attack, and help ameliorate intestinal disorders.

What's the verdict on yogurt?

The case against yogurt. Regular plain yogurt is about 50% fat, expressed in terms of total calories. That's about the same as whole milk. But yogurt has somewhat more cholesterol than whole milk (more than 3.5% by weight). Calories contributed by milk and yogurt are about the same, and in both cases most of the calories come from saturated fats. When flavorings and preserves are added to yogurt, it has considerably more calories than whole milk—and most of the added calories come from sugar. Some yogurts are artificially colored, and contain additives.

Yogurt has less vitamins A and C than milk; and, far from being an ideal food, provides quantities of iron, copper, and vitamin C below government Required Daily Allowances. If the yogurt is pasteurized, the bacteria are killed off, and the product has no therapeutic value.

If you have a choice of a 244-calorie lunch of tuna with tomato and lettuce, followed by a peach and a glass of milk, or a 170-calorie lunch of strawberry yogurt, you would be better off nutritionally with the tuna lunch, according to Consumers Union (the extra 74 calories will have virtually no effect on your weight). "A very expensive glass of milk," is what Consumers Union calls yogurt.

The case for yogurt. Yogurt has a greater content of potassium, phosphorus, and zinc than milk, more protein, and higher levels of vitamin B_{12} and folic acid. It is more easily digested than milk. If you drink a quart or more of yogurt a day, it could lower blood-cholesterol levels significantly, and help block the cholesterol pathway to heart attack. Some evidence indicates that yogurt can speed the recovery of patients suffering from diarrhea caused by antibiotics; and yogurt generally will not aggravate the condition of persons afflicted with intestinal disorders.

The verdict. On balance, yogurt appears to be a high-fat, high saturated-fat, but otherwise nutritious, food, holding out some promise of health-promoting qualities. I don't use regular yogurt.

But I do use the plain low-fat variety, which has only 24% fat in terms of total calories, because of its health possibilities and its culinary actualities. Yogurt adds bite and creaminess to low-fat cottage cheese, piquancy to some of my breads, and the proper touch of the exotic to my dishes derived from the great cuisines of India and the Near and Middle East. Mixed with naturally sweet fruit, and accented with sweet spices, yogurt makes a low-calorie dessert as refreshing as it is delectable.

Non-fat milk. I use a low-heat-process non-fat dry milk which is not instantized. Instant dry milk is made by rewetting the dried solids, a process which impairs the natural flavor. Blended or shaken with spring water, the non-instant solid reconstitutes into a delicious, fresh-tasting milk with no loss of flavor.

This non-fat milk has the same percentages of vitamins and minerals (particularly calcium) as whole milk. Fat is almost zero per cup (less than 1 gram), which produces a 90-calorie-a-cup milk (whole milk has about 160 calories a cup).

For use in decaffeinated coffee or in coffee taste-alikes, prepare double strength. Dry or reconstituted, it's an admirable replacement for whole milk in cooking.

Buttermilk. Despite its name, buttermilk, which is produced from the whey in the butter-making process, is as low in calories and fat as low-fat milk. If you like its sourish taste (I do), it makes a refreshing cold drink. It adds a provocative sharpness to many of my entrées, and something elusively different to my breads. Be sure the label reads: "No salt added."

Don't use synthetic dairy products, such as imitation sour cream, whipped toppings, non-dairy creamers, and butter substitutes. Aside from their plethora of chemical non-food ingredients, these ersatz foods are loaded with highly saturated coconut and palm oils.

You Can't Cook without Oil

Oil transmits and enhances the flavors of other ingredients. It adds savor and crispness to skillet dishes, smoothness and body to salad

dressings, and clingyness to marinades. Dry-skillet cooking and sautéing in water or broth are sad substitutes for sautéing with oil.

Cooking with oil makes nutritional, as well as culinary, sense. All
cooking oils are vegetable, so there's nary a trace of cholesterol in
any of them, and they're high in polyunsaturated fats. (But beware
of hydrogenated vegetable oils; they're partially or completely saturated.) Vegetable oils help supply the body with essential vitamins,
minerals, and fatty acids; and they aid in the absorption of fat-
soluble vitamins A, D, E, and K. Vegetable oils are easily digestible.

The Gourmet Fat-Conscious Shopper's Guide to Cooking and Salad Oils

All oils are 100% fat. (An oil is a fat which is liquid at room
temperature.) From a health standpoint, oils high in polyunsaturated fats are preferred. The following guide provides the ratio of
polyunsaturated fats to saturated fats (P:S) in oils available in supermarkets, health-food stores, and gourmet shops.

A P:S ratio of 1:1 (peanut oil) means there's as much polyunsaturated fat in the oil as saturated fat. A P:S ratio of 7:1 (safflower oil)
means the oil contains 7 times as much polyunsaturated fat as saturated fat. A P:S ratio of trace:1 means the oil is virtually all saturated fat.

Here are the P:S values of fats and oils forbidden *on the Diet for
Life:*

Oil	P:S
Avocado oil	trace:1
Beef fat	1:5
Butter	trace:1
Chicken fat	1:5
Coconut oil	trace:1
Egg yolk*	1:5
Lamb fat	trace:1
Lard	trace:1
Margarines (partially hydrogenated)	1:1.2
Palm oil	trace:1
Peanut oil	1:1
Vegetable shortenings (hydrogenated)	trace:1 to 1:1

* Permissible only in small quantities.

Here are the P:S values of oils acceptable *on the Diet for Life:*

Oil	P:S
Almond oil	4:1
All-purpose oil	4:1
Apricot-kernel oil	5:1
Corn oil	4.5:1
Cottonseed oil	1.6:1
Margarines	
tub: liquid safflower	5.1:1
tub: liquid corn oil	2.7:1
stick: liquid corn oil	2:1
imitation (diet)	2.5:1
Olive oil	1.4:1
Safflower oil	7:1
Sesame oil	3:1
Soybean oil	4.3:1
(lightly hydrogenated)	2.4:1
Sunflower oil	5.3:1
Walnut oil	4.5:1

FAT-WISE HINTS ABOUT OILS

- *Comforting note:* unsaturated fats are not converted to saturated fats when heated to high cooking temperatures.
- Cold-pressed oil is preferred to oils extracted by steam or chemicals, both of which spoil flavor and undermine nutritional values. Oils from the first pressing—virgin oils—are top-quality buys.
- Oils with high smoking points are best for cooking. All oils begin to smoke—reach their smoking points—at different temperatures. Beyond the smoking point, the oil decomposes, becoming ugly to look at and repulsive to the palate. Acceptable oils with high smoking points are corn and cottonseed. (I rule out cottonseed, though, on the basis of its lackluster taste.) Oils with low smoking points should be limited to salad dressings.
- Corn oil predominates in my recipes because of its high P:S ratio of 4.5:1; it's light, buttery corn flavor; its perfect blendship with other ingredients of salad dressings and marinades; its high smoking point; and its wide availability and budget price. Vegetable oils with equal or higher P:S ratios have none of the other qualities.
- Here's a rundown on the taste characteristics of popular vegetable oils other than corn. *Safflower oil* is flavorless, and greasy to the point of repugnance in salads. *Soybean oil* is insipid. *Cottonseed oil* has nothing to recommend it. On the other hand, *sesame oil,* with its distinctive nutty flavor, can be mixed with corn oil to add distinction to salad dressings and sautéed foods; and *olive oil*—that incomparable oil—can

be blended likewise to add excitement to everything it touches. (Olive oil, because of its fairly low P:S ratio of 1.4:1, should only be used blended in small quantities with oils of considerably higher P:S ratios.)

· Oils can go bad, even on a store shelf, when exposed to heat and/or strong light. You'll know when it's gone bad by its rancid odor. I keep my unopened containers of oil in a cool, dark cupboard, and my opened containers in my refrigerator. Under refrigeration, the corn oil I use lasts for weeks without loss of flavor. If the oil you use solidifies under refrigeration (my corn oil doesn't), simply restore it to room temperature and the oil will liquefy. Solidification (freezing) does not alter the nutritional qualities or the original flavor of oil.

· Never store oil in a plastic container. An unhappy chemical reaction takes place that distorts the natural character of the oil. A glass container, particularly if it's light-resistant, preserves the original attractiveness of the oil longer.

· I use margarine judiciously, in both cooking and as a spread. If you do use margarine, determine the P:S ratio by dividing grams of polyunsaturated fats by grams of saturated fats as listed on the label, and select the margarine with the highest ratio. Be sure no salt has been added.

What About Cholesterol?

Cholesterol is not, as most people think, a lethal fat. It's a sterol—a waxy alcohol—and leads a Jekyll-and-Hyde existence.

Cholesterol maintains the health of the body in several important ways. It's the insulating sheath for the delicate neural electrical system. It strengthens the membranes which control what goes in and out of every cell of the body. It makes digestion possible by helping in the manufacture of bile acids. And it's a building block for such hormones as progesterone, which governs the menstrual cycle, and relatives of adrenaline, which powers the body in times of stress.

On the other hand, cholesterol can turn itself into tough, tiny crystalline spears which can embed themselves into the walls of the cardiovascular system, trapping fat particles, cellular debris, and possibly calcium deposits to form a layer of plaque which narrows the arteries. As the plaque grows, like an encrustation on the inside of a pipe, the flow of blood to the heart is reduced to a trickle; and some of the heart, or all of it, starved for oxygen carried in the blood, shuts down partially or completely. That's a heart attack.

The body has a built-in device for keeping the arteries clear of cholesterol: high-density lipoproteins (H.D.L.'s). A lipoprotein is a combination of a protein and a fat (lipid); and there's another kind in the bloodstream beside H.D.L.'s. Low-density lipoproteins (L.D.P.'s) carry cholesterol to the sites in the body where it's needed (cholesterol is not soluble in water and cannot be carried by the

254

bloodstream as such). When there's an excess of cholesterol, it's likely that the L.D.L.'s dump some of their load onto the arterial walls. The H.D.L.'s then clear out the deposits like a Roto-Rooter, and carry off the excess cholesterol for eventual elimination. We're born with equal amounts of L.D.L.'s and H.D.L.'s, but mainly through nutritional abuse of our bodies, L.D.L.'s in adult life outnumber H.D.L.s by a factor as high as seven. A sound nutritional program should bring that factor down to at least three or four.

Since the body can manufacture its own cholesterol, banning all cholesterol from the diet seems to make sense. But no one knows if the body makes sufficient cholesterol to satisfy its needs; an optimal amount of ingested cholesterol may be necessary. Prudently, some investigators have established a safety zone for cholesterol consumption of 160-185 milligrams a day. (Most Americans consume about 800 milligrams a day.) Below that zone, cholesterol deprivation is suspected. Above it, redundant cholesterol may overburden the L.D.L.'s and start the process of plaque formation. On the Diet for Life, we stay within the cholesterol safety zone.

But there is a great body of evidence leading to the conclusion that ingested cholesterol does not contribute to pathological levels of blood cholesterol, and consequently cannot be a cause of heart attack. That should delight egg lovers, since a single egg yolk contains 250 milligrams of cholesterol, far more than the cholesterol-safety-zone maximum of 185 milligrams a day. Because of the ambiguity concerning the harmful effects of ingested cholesterol, and because eggs are magnificently nutritious, two eggs a week spaced days apart are included on the Diet for Life as an option for egg lovers. But if you want to play it safe, eat half a yolk each time. And if you want to play it even safer (as we do), eat only the egg white. But *don't* opt for egg substitutes. They're about 50% fattier than eggs, and are synthesized mainly from non-nutrient chemicals.

Here is a list of—

HIGH-CHOLESTEROL FOODS TO BE AVOIDED

(Arranged in ascending order of cholesterol content. Three ounces uncooked is equivalent to four ounces cooked. Cholesterol is given in milligrams.)

Food	Cholesterol (mg.)
Lard, 1 cup	208
Eggs, 1 yolk or 1 egg	250 *
Cream, whipping, 1 cup	316
Liver (beef, calf, hog, or lamb), 3 ounces cooked	372

*See preceding paragraph.

Butter, whipped, 1 cup	380
Sweetbreads, 3 ounces cooked	396
Pork spareribs, 3 ounces cooked	516
Butter, regular, 1 cup	564
Duck, 3 ounces cooked	660
Kidneys, 3 ounces cooked	680
Brains, 3 ounces cooked	2,675

But some foods popularly regarded as high in cholesterol do fall within the cholesterol safety zone when eaten in moderate-sized portions that do not push the day's caloric intake over the 185-milligram permissible maximum. Here is a list of—

"HIGH"-CHOLESTEROL FOODS YOU CAN LIVE WITH

(Arranged in ascending order of cholesterol content. Three ounces uncooked is equivalent to four ounces cooked. Cholesterol is given in milligrams.)

Food	Cholesterol (mg.)
Oysters, 3 ounces cooked	40
Salmon, 3 ounces cooked	40
Scallops, 3 ounces cooked	45
Clams, 3 ounces cooked	55
Tuna, 3 ounces cooked	55
Halibut, 3 ounces cooked	55
Swordfish, 3 ounces cooked	63
Pork (other than spareribs) 3 ounces cooked	75
Beef, 3 ounces cooked	75
Lobster, 3 ounces cooked	75
Poultry, dark meat; 3 ounces cooked	75
Lamb, 3 ounces cooked	85
Crab, 3 ounces cooked	85
Cheese, 3 ounces	90
Shrimp, 11 large	96
Sardines, 3 ounces cooked	130

You'll find no cholesterol in vegetables, fruits, grains, nuts, seeds, and wines.

PART FOUR

Vitamins, Minerals, and Exercise Help You Live Your Life to the Fullest

13

Forgetting What Fatigue Feels Like—and Feeling Fully Alive

We begin our day with a vitamin cocktail. The recipe is simple: four ounces of apple juice (no sugar added), fresh lime juice to taste, plus a dozen vitamins. On an empty stomach, the natural sugars from the fruit juices surge swiftly into the bloodstream, giving us that "Oh, what a wonderful morning!" feeling. And the vitamins, tuning up each cell of the body to peak efficiency, help propel us through the morning with high energy.

All the healthful food in the Diet for Life would be wasted if it were not supplemented with vitamins. Vitamins are nutrients—not drugs, even though they are purchased in capsules—which transmute the food we eat into living tissue and living energy. Deprived of vitamins for some length of time, cells deteriorate, even die. Vitamin-deficiency diseases—like scurvy (lack of vitamin C), rickets (lack of vitamin D), and night blindness (lack of vitamin A)—have long been scourges of the world's undernourished.

Few Americans suffer from these diseases. Our national diet, woefully inadequate in so many other aspects, supplies vitamins in sufficient quantities to forestall pathological breakdowns. But those quantities are not sufficient to keep the cells in our body operating at more than minimal efficiency. Each cell struggles through the day like an assembly-line worker with one hand tied behind his back, working many times harder just to get by. The result is that tired, dragged-out feeling. The strain of fatigue, day in and day out, wears down the body; and you're beset by vague and fleeting aches and pains, listlessness, lack of endurance, and a general feeling of poor health.

Why Your Food Is Vitamin-Poor

What happens to your food on the way to your kitchen is one reason why vitamins come to you in short supply. Processing destroys virtually all vitamins (and the vitamins are restored in only a few kinds of food). Even unprocessed food arrives deficient in vitamins. Fruits are plucked green, vegetables are harvested before they're ripe—and vitamin production is halted long before the full quota has been reached. In transit, usually over long distances, foods are exposed to heat, light, cold, shocks—all vitamin-destructive traumas. The vitamin C value of a potato can drop 1,000% by the time you're ready to eat it.

Whatever vitamin content remains in your food when you bring it home from the supermarket is further eroded in your kitchen. The chemical structures of vitamins crumble in poorly sealed containers, and when exposed to light; and they disintegrate when thawed slowly after refrigeration. As you cut, pare, and peel, the vitamins in the flesh of the food are exposed to attack by the oxygen in the air. Cooking heat breaks down most of the vitamins, and re-heating virtually finishes the destruction that heating began. A delay in serving, while oxidation plays havoc with the heated food, could wipe out any stray vitamins that remain.

Even if you could protect your food from vitamin depredation every step of the way from shopping cart to dining-room table, you still couldn't be sure how much of the certified vitamin content would go to work for you. Some enriched breakfast cereals, for example, do supply a full day's supply of vitamins necessary to prevent vitamin-deficiency diseases; but often vitamin B_3 is present in a form which cannot be metabolized. And while charts show an ample supply of vitamins in carrots, much of it is contained in cells your body can't break into.

Because your food is vitamin-poor (and also because you're robbed of vitamins by smoking, pollution, alcohol, oral contraceptives, and stress)—

Vitamin Supplements Are Necessary

Vitamins work together as a team, so you need supplements of all of them. The quantities you need are ordinarily greater than the U.S. R.D.A.'s—the United States Recommended Daily Allowances—for vitamins set by the federal Food and Drug Administration (F.D.A.) based on recommendations of the National Research Council of the National Academy of Sciences. U.S. R.D.A.'s for vitamins are sufficiently high to ward off deficiency diseases, but not always high enough to help ensure peak energy.

How to Determine Your Vitamin Supplement Requirements for Maximum Energy

The amounts of each vitamin supplement necessary to help you operate at your top energy level—your Dynamic Daily Allowance, your D.D.A. rather than your R.D.A.—must be determined by yourself. There are no standards because everyone has different requirements. Finding yours is a matter of trial and error. Here's how Harold found his.

He started with R.D.A.'s for vitamins C, D, E, and the B complex. He increased his dosage of vitamin C by 100 milligrams a week. There's no way to test energy levels, but you can feel changes in energy, and week by week Harold felt his energy levels rising. At 4,300 milligrams, he felt no further energy increase. He cut back to 4,200 milligrams. That's his D.D.A. for vitamin C.

He then followed the same procedure for each of the other vitamins in turn, increasing weekly dosage by the smallest available commercial unit, until one week's dosage no longer produced a subjective energy increment. The dosage for the preceding week became his D.D.A. Here are Harold's D.D.A.'s compared with his R.D.A.'s for the 15 vitamins he takes daily.

ONE ADULT'S
DYNAMIC DAILY ALLOWANCE FOR VITAMINS

Vitamin	D.D.A.'s	R.D.A.'s
A (retinol)	10,000 I.U.	5,000 I.U.*
D (cholecalciferol)	400 I.U.	400 I.U.*
E (alpha tocopherol)	1,200 I.U.	30 I.U.*
C (ascorbic acid)	4,200 mg.	60 mg.
The B-complex vitamins		
B_1 (thiamin)	50 mg.	1.5 mg.
B_2 (riboflavin)	50 mg.	1.7 mg.
B_3 (niacin)	50 mg.	20 mg.
B_6 (pyridoxine)	50 mg.	2 mg.
B_{12} (cobalamin)	50 mcg.	6 mcg.
Pantothenic acid (anti-stress vitamin)	50 mg.	10 mg
Folic acid (folacin)	400 mcg.	400 mcg.
Biotin (vitamin H)	300 mcg.	300 mcg.
Choline	50 mcg.	None
Inositol	50 mcg.	None
PABA (Para aminobenzoic acid)	50 mg.	None

NOTE: I.U. = International Units; mg. = milligrams; mcg. = micrograms ($\frac{1}{1,000}$ of a milligram)

---

* Vitamins A, D, and E are expressed in terms of I.U.'s for easy comparison with the I.U.'s on the labels of our vitamin bottles. The 1980 U.S. R.D.A.'s for these vitamins are not expressed as I.U.'s, but as follows: A (retinol equivalents), 400; D (mcg. of cholecalciferol), 5; E (mg. alpha-tocopherol equivalents), 10.

Vitamin K doesn't appear on the list because intestinal bacteria produce it in sufficient quantities from Diet for Life edibles which include beef, pork, leafy vegetables, tomatoes, peas, and cauliflower. (Besides, in excessive quantities vitamin K is toxic.) Also excluded is the officially unrecognized vitamin B_{15} (pangamic acid). Despite evidence from abroad which invests it with a Lourdes-like aura (it's claimed to cure everything from allergies to senility), we rejected it because even in small quantities it gave Harold arthritic-like aches in the shoulder muscles. The symptoms ceased as soon as vitamin B_{15} was dropped.

Included on the list are two vitamins which have not been recognized by the F.D.A.: inositol and PABA. A preponderance of evidence places them among the vitamins of the B complex.

I take the same 15 vitamins as Harold, but C and E in different quantities. Using Harold's procedure, I gradually upped my vitamin C intake to a D.D.A. of 3,000 milligrams, and my vitamin E intake to 800 I.U.

Both of us are aware there are reports of pathological effects of large dosages of vitamins. Beyond 10,000 I.U.'s a day, vitamin A can stop menstruation; destroy bone; cause headaches, abdominal pain, nausea, profuse sweating, and jaundice; and destroy blood cells. Large doses of vitamin C have resulted in diarrhea, destruction of B_{12}, loss of calcium from bones, and the formation of bladder and kidney stones. Excessive consumption of vitamin D can damage the kidney, and induce lethargy and loss of appetite. Overdoses of vitamin E have brought on hypertension, headache, nausea, extreme fatigue, and muscle weakness.

At the first sign of any of these symptoms, or of any persistent unpleasant symptoms associated with augmented vitamin ingestion, cut back on your intake of the offending vitamin at once.

Warning: when considering the use of vitamin supplements, or a change in the amounts of your regular supplements, it is wise to seek the advice of your physician.

Vitamins Help You Feel Fully Alive . . .

. . . because they're carriers of health. No vitamin can operate at its full potential without the presence of all others, but in teams of several vitamins, and individually, they operate in specific ways to keep the body healthy.

As teams, vitamins A, C, and D bring health to the skeletal system; B_1, B_3, and B_6 to the intestines; B_1, B_3, C, choline, E, and inositol, to the cardiovascular system; B_1, B_2, biotin, E, folic acid, K, and PABA, to the blood; B_1, B_3, B_6, B_{12}, folic acid, and pantothenic acid, to the nervous system; A, B_1, B_2, B_3, C, D, and K, to the eyes; and A, B_2, B_3, B_6, biotin, C, and K, to the skin.

As individuals, vitamins function in the following major ways:

Vitamin E is necessary, among other things, for the metabolism of polyunsaturated fats. (On the Diet for Life, the majority of the fat is polyunsaturated, and an adequate supply of vitamin E is important.) Vitamin C, among its other activities, stimulates the immune system which fights bacterial and viral invaders. (Since we've been on high dosages of vitamin C, 4,200 milligrams a day for Harold and 3,000 for me, neither of us has had a single cold. At the slightest hint of a cold, we take an additional 1,000 milligrams each hour until the pre-symptoms disappear. That takes from two to six hours.)

Both vitamins C and E are associated with resistance to degenerative diseases. Both are also antioxidants, chemicals which retard cellular aging. (Harold looks at least 10 years younger than he is, and people always guess my age to be flatteringly young.) Vitamins C and E are also effective against pollutants and some cancer-causing chemicals.

Vitamin A helps fight air pollutants by maintaining a strong line of defense in the mucous membranes of tear ducts and respiratory organs. We look to vitamin A, as well as the vitamins of the B complex (especially in combination with vitamin C), to combat stress, which may be the foremost non-nutritive cause of disease of our time. Vitamin D is relied upon to cut our dental bills, and to maintain a youthful skeletal structure (we won't bend or shrink as we grow older). And we employ choline and inositol as scouring agents to help cleanse the arteries of cholesterol deposits.

Of vital importance, also, in maintaining the health of the body, and the feeling of being fully alive that accompanies it, are the essential minerals, including the trace elements—micro-nutrients which are required in extremely small amounts. Unlike vitamins, these inorganic compounds are hardy, and, by and large, remain intact in sufficient quantities in food despite the abuses of processing, shipping, storing, cooking, and serving. (When minerals are removed in processing, they're usually replaced in adequate amounts in the marketed products.) In your food and water, you can get your required Daily Allowances of all the minerals you need, with the possible exception of iron. If you're in normal health, you don't need mineral supplements. In fact—

Mineral Supplements Can Be Toxic

In large quantities, here's what essential minerals can do to you. Copper can poison you, as can iodine, silicon, vanadium, tin, nickel, and molybdenum. Zinc can cause severe anemia, abdominal pain, fever, nausea, and vomiting. Fluorine can mottle your teeth. Cobalt can induce heart-muscle damage, a blood disease, and goiter. Manganese can blur your speech, give you a permanent deadpan expression, send tremors through your hands, make walking difficult, and bring on involuntary laughter. Selenium can attack the teeth and nervous system.

More iron than you need can induce hemochromatosis, which can damage the liver, pancreas, and heart; and increase the likelihood and severity of fungus and bacterial infections since iron is a preferred food of these microorganisms. But, according to a recent scientific study, many Americans have less to fear from excess iron than from iron deficiency, which is the most common cause of anemia. "Tired blood" is iron-deficiency anemia.

What to Do About "Tired Blood"

When there's not enough iron in the blood (in the form of a compound called hemoglobin), insufficient oxygen is carried to the tissues, causing weakness, lack of stamina, pallor, and shortness of breath. About 5% of the women in this country suffer from this type of anemia. Blood tests can reveal an anemic condition; and iron supplements taken under medical supervision can help restore normalcy.

Harold and I rely on natural sources for our iron: potatoes, salad greens, dried beans and peas, fresh and dried apricots, raisins, walnuts, pork and beef, oysters, enriched cereals, and apples. Other excellent iron sources—kidneys, egg yolks, and liver—are high in cholesterol, and are to be avoided. So is blackstrap molasses, another excellent iron source, because it has a high sucrose content. Spinach, despite Popeye and popular opinion, is not a good source of iron, because the leaf contains oxalates which hinder iron absorption.

An old-fashioned do-it-yourself way to enrich foods with iron is to cook in an iron pot. Iron from the pot is absorbed by the food. The current epidemic of mild anemia—it's the country's most widespread nutritional-deficiency disease—may have been caused in part by the large-scale switchover to non-stick-surface cookware. (Since our diet is naturally iron-rich, I take advantage of non-stick cookware to cut fat consumption. Even if you're watching your fat consumption, you can use an iron skillet on occasion provided you employ minimum amounts of oil and keep heat low enough to prevent sticking.)

But even when iron is ingested in sufficient quantities, it may not be utilized by the body when certain foods are eaten which obstruct iron absorption. Spinach, milk, egg whites, and tea are the most powerful of these anti-absorbents; and I eliminate them during my period, when I'm intensely aware of the need for iron. At that time of the month, I eat more beef, fish, and poultry because their iron content is absorbed easily. (If you're not watching cholesterol, add liver to that list.) Absorption of iron from any source at any time of the month is heightened by the use of vitamin C supplements (only 25 milligrams can increase iron absorption by as much as 50%).

What About Mineral Waters?

We get our R.D.A. of essential minerals from our Diet for Life foods (Chapter 9) and from spring water. We prefer spring water to tap water not because of its superior mineral content (New York City tap water can match or surpass most spring waters in that respect), but because of its taste and the absence of unwanted additives. We won't touch distilled water, which has been stripped of its minerals, and bears the same relationship to wholesome water as empty calories do to wholesome food.

Mineral waters contain more minerals than most spring waters, and in greater quantities. Since mineral supplements are usually not necessary, except perhaps for iron, there's no nutritional advantage in consuming mineral waters. But other than in the U.S.A., mineral waters are extolled for their powers to cure almost everything from flatulence to corpulence; and their attractiveness lies in their purported health-promoting qualities. Of those properties, two have been verified: some mineral waters are potent laxatives; and some others are useful anti-acids (they're the waters labeled "alkaline"). In this country, making a therapeutic claim for a mineral water is against the law.

On occasions, for the taste alone, we enjoy Perrier with or without a slice of lime (but never during meals). It's low in sodium, as are Evian and Mountain Valley. We turn our back, though, on Saratoga, Vichy Céléstin, and San Pellegrino, because their sodium content is on the high side. There are some 30 brands of mineral waters marketed in this country, and it would be wise to label-check for sodium before quaffing. Search the labels, too, for lithium. It's one of the most prescribed drugs in the psychiatrist's pharmacopeia; but the effect consistent ingestion will have on you if you're not mentally disturbed has not been explored.

Healthful food, D.D.A.'s of vitamins, and R.D.A.'s of essential minerals are the nutritional ingredients for a peak energy. On the Diet for Life, they're combined in—

Meal and Snack Patterns to Keep Your Energy
High All Day Long

If the engines of a 747 were to be fueled erratically, the jet could not sustain its power thrust, speed would be cut drastically, and the plane would be in danger of crashing. Much like the 747, the human body needs a constant energy supply to keep it flying high. But while fuel is pumped into jet engines steadily, we feed our bodies only three to five times a day (three meals and one or two snacks). Each time we eat, we must pattern our food selection in such a way that the proper balance of carbohydrates, proteins, fats, vitamins, and minerals produces a fairly constant flow of energy which will endure from one eating time to the next.

Here are Diet For Life meal and snack patterns:

Pre-breakfast snack. Just as the 747 requires a sudden surge of energy to lift it off the runway, we need a pick-me-up to start our day. It's the vitamin cocktail I introduced you to at the beginning of this chapter. The vitamins are the water solubles: vitamin C (about 40% of our D.D.A.) and the 11 vitamins of the B complex (100% of our D.D.A.). There's no fat in this snack, so no fat-soluble vitamins are included in this cocktail. The body will draw on its stored fat-soluble vitamins until lunch. The fruit juices contain a plethora of minerals.

Enjoy this pre-breakfast snack—it's as sharp, cold, and invigorating as an autumn morning—just as soon as you get out of bed. Then when you look into your bathroom mirror, you'll see an eager face, glowing with vitality, ready to take on the world. The cocktail will refresh your taste buds, arouse your sleep-dulled appetite, and you'll approach your breakfast table with a sense of anticipatory joy. It's a terrific way to start the day!

Breakfast. If you're like many weight-conscious Americans, you make the deplorable mistake of beginning your day with just a cup of coffee. The caffeine gives you a lift for a short time, then crashes you into depression, nervousness, irritability, and exhaustion. You need another lift, so, another cup; but that lets you down, too; and you need another cup, and another cup and another; and you're trapped into a cycle of caffeine highs and lows all day long. You ride an emotional pogo stick, shaking up your nervous system, and shattering your sense of well-being.

It makes sense to break the coffee habit, and get into the breakfast habit. A sound breakfast can give you a better high than coffee, and keep you high until lunch (you don't need that coffee break and that high-caloric Danish that goes with it). It's a different kind of high: it soothes your nerves instead of jangling them; it makes you feel calmly wonderful, instead of all hopped up. It's a food high, not a drug high—and that's the distinction between health and hype.

The food pattern for a Diet for Life breakfast consists of mainly complex carbohydrates, supported by some protein and some simple carbohydrates. The complex carbohydrates come from cereals, bread, and rolls; the protein from non-fat milk and egg whites; and the simple carbohydrates from fresh, dried, and cooked fruits, and honey. There's a plentitude of minerals in these foods. You've already taken your morning's vitamin supplements.

The simple carbohydrates (sugar) in the fruits and honey will give you an instant lift, and the complex carbohydrates and protein, metabolizing slowly, will keep your energy and your spirits high all morning long.

Breakfast is the most important meal of the day. Prove it by looking into your mirror at 10 A.M. of a breakfastless day and at the same time on a day in which you enjoyed a Diet for Life breakfast. On your breakfastless day, your face looks fallen and old. On your breakfast day, it's firm and youthful. Nutritional face lift! It reflects your uplifted spirits. Breakfast energy gives you the emotional power to help deal with the challenges of the morning ahead—and that could make you feel better about yourself all day. Don't ever start a day without breakfast—a Diet for Life breakfast.

Lunch. On a breakfastless day, even when you indulge yourself during the coffee break, midday is food-madness time. You gobble up everything in front of you, and still want more. But fortified with a Diet for Life breakfast, noontime is light-eating time. Your breakfast nutrients have been consumed slowly, and as noon approaches, your blood-sugar level edges gently into the hunger zone. There's no compulsion to overeat, and a small amount of food soon elevates your blood sugar, and your body's STOP! eating signal flashes.

At lunch, fat joins the food pattern. There's a longer interval between lunch and dinner than between breakfast and lunch (sometimes as much as four hours); and lunch foods must supply long-lasting energy. It can't be done without fat, which is metabolized more slowly than other nutrients. The dominant Diet for Life fat is highly polyunsaturated corn oil; and I use it at lunch in my salad dressings, and mixed into many enticing leftover creations. About 40% of the Diet for Life's daily fat allowance goes into my lunch dishes.

Our protein for lunch comes mainly from tinned salt-free fish, egg whites, and leftover meat, fish, and poultry. Our complex carbohydrates are derived for the most part from salad greens, raw vegetables, and bread and rolls. Our simple carbohydrates, which quickly zoom energy levels back to their morning highs, are obtained from fresh or dried fruit, and fruit juices.

Contrary to most dieters' opinions, fresh fruit salad makes a poor luncheon dish. Its glut of simple carbohydrates is used up so fast that you're hungry again in a short time. When we do have a fruit salad for lunch, we add low-fat cottage cheese (protein) and a salad dressing (fat). But even then we know we'll need a snack about 4 or 5 in the afternoon.

Fat-soluble vitamins E (50% of our D.D.A.) and A and D (100% of our D.D.A.), as well as another increment of vitamin C (about 20% of our D.D.A.), are taken immediately after lunch. The fat-soluble vitamins are included in the lunch pattern because the meal provides sufficient fat to dissolve them; and more vitamin C is necessary because the body utilizes this nutrient rapidly. Our luncheon food is replete with minerals.

More afternoon energy comes from exercise (more about that later in the chapter) and from rest. Harold walks after lunch and then siestas. I can't nap (strangely, most men can, and most women can't), and I envy him. In Rome, where the siesta has been a custom since antiquity, most of the population is certain that dozing off at midday keeps the heart young, adds years to your life, stimulates sexual desire, and refreshes you mentally and physically for the second part of your workday. Judging from Harold, when at home, do as the Romans do.

Late-afternoon snack. There are times when we're working hard, or when we've had a fresh fruit salad for lunch, that we feel the need for a picker-upper around 4 in the afternoon. A small amount of raisins and walnuts does the job: raisins (simple carbohydrates) to restore the energy level fast; and walnuts (polyunsaturated fat) to keep those levels high for the rest of the afternoon. Any combination of a simple-carbohydrate source (dried fruits) and a rich polyunsaturated source (almonds, seeds) can be enjoyed, as well. Just remember: it's a snack, not a *meal.*

Dinner. This is our largest meal of the day. Three reasons:

The first reason is emotional. The day's work is done, and we want to relax at length over the delights of the table. In our household, dinner has always been a time of peace and serenity, of sharing, of conviviality. Dinner time is like a book you love so much you never want it to end.

The other reasons are biological. Evening is meant for letting down, taking it easy, readying the body for sleep. The light meals you've had during the day supply just enough calories to speed you up, but the increased amount of calories in the evening meal slows you down. You still have sufficient energy to enjoy your evening's leisure—go out, dance, bowl, read, watch TV, converse, make love— but sleep is on its way, and the pace of the body decelerates pleasantly.

After dinner, it will be 12 long hours or so before you eat again, and you need a storehouse of food upon which to draw. And that's the third reason for the larger evening meal: it has to sustain you until you break your fast in the morning.

Dinner, then, is the time for higher-calorie, stick-to-the-ribs foods; and protein and fat dominate. We eat protein-rich meat, fish, and poultry, garnering their natural fats. I prepare my dishes with corn oil, sometimes accented with olive oil; and my salad dressings would be incomplete without oil. The carbohydrates are for the most part complex: salad greens and cooked vegetables; potatoes, rice, and kasha; pies, cookies, and cakes. Not infrequently we have wine—a food, not an empty calorie—and the queen of relaxants.

After dinner, the remainder of our D.D.A.'s for vitamins are consumed; and in concert with the profusion of minerals from our evening meal, they continue to maintain our cells at peak efficiency while we sleep. The activity of the cells is low, for rest is necessary for reinvigoration; but throughout the night each cell purrs with latent energy. In the morning when we awaken from a blissful, unbroken slumber, we're ready to go. Our pre-breakfast vitamin cocktail gets us started.

Then during the day, we boost the energy derived from food with exercise.

Walk Your Way to Greater Vitality

There's no question about the salutary effects of exercise. But our life is built around the pleasure principle: if you don't enjoy it, it won't do you any good; and most exercises rate from boring to painful. I have never seen a happy jogger. We exercise as we eat, joyfully, with the oldest exercise known to mankind—walking.

We don't set out with a pedometer, and hike X miles a day at the rate of Y miles an hour carrying a load of Z pounds. Where's the joy in that? We walk when we have to go someplace, when we crave solitude, when we need the stimulation of fresh sights and sounds, when we want to talk things over, when we desire to feel the wind in our hair. Walking is part of our life.

Walking energizes. Unlike other exercises, it doesn't leave you exhausted. It's so invigorating, you can actually walk fatigue away. I've seen a work-burdened Harold come back after a two-mile walk with color in his cheeks, eyes shining, and sit down at his typewriter for five to six hours in a row. Walking gives you stamina and endurance, and a zest for carrying on.

Walking is a tonic for the spirit. You come away from a walk relaxed, composed, at ease; anger, tension, depression, frustration—gone. Walking is nature's tranquilizer. As you walk, your thoughts flow. How often have I unraveled a knotty problem as I strode through the city streets! When you walk alone with your mind free, daydreams flourish. When you walk with a companion, friendship flourishes, and even love. Men and women don't jog down lovers' lane; they walk—hand in hand.

The body responds to walking with a healthful glow, because nature intended us to walk. Sit or stand for some time, and your back aches, your muscles and joints stiffen, your neck and shoulders droop with fatigue. But walking builds and loosens muscles, and replaces tiredness and pain with a sense of vitality and well-being.

Walking reduces blood pressure, helps cleanse blood of harmful triglycerides, boosts the levels of cholesterol-scavenging H.D.L.'s, unglues sticky blood that can clot into a thrombosis, and increases the flow of blood to the heart. Stroll, saunter, or stride, and you counter the loss of calcium from bones, the scourge that shrinks the skeletal structure of women after menopause. Walking can prevent the replacement of muscle tissue by fat, fight headaches, and even retard some of the symptoms of old age. Walking can help ward off disease, and help rehabilitate the body after disease has struck.

Walking is an aid to weight control. Walk three miles in an hour daily, and in three weeks you can drop a pound without dropping a calorie. You'll look trimmer than the non-walker of the same weight, because walking builds muscle tissue, and muscle tissue occupies less volume than fat. Walking makes you look younger and sexier.

And walking is safe (unless your doctor tells you it's not; an orthopedic problem or a chronic illness may restrain you). With strenuous excercise, you face the chance of injury. Several deaths have occurred shortly after jogging. But if you're healthy, there's little risk from walking; and walking is medically prescribed for some sufferers from emphysema, heart disease, diabetes, and arthritis.

If you're a beginner, keep in mind that the backs of your legs are likely to tighten up. Loosen them by stretching. Walk a little farther each day. In no time at all, walking will become, as nature meant it to be, first nature to you.

One last advantage: you need no special equipment, no health spa, no swimming pool, no instructors, no uniform—no bucks. It's cheap!

Get out and walk!

We work very hard—I've seen Harold put in 14-hour workdays, seven days a week, for weeks in a row; and I'm always hard at work in the kitchen, writing new recipes, shopping for ingredients, and researching new nutritional data—but we've forgotten what fatigue feels like. Our formula for peak energy is this: the Diet for Life—healthful food brimming with minerals, supplemented by the quantities of vitamins right for you—plus walking as a part of your life.

And as your energy peaks, you'll get a feeling of joy, of excitement, of pulsating power—a feeling of wanting to do wonderful things, and of knowing that you can do them—a feeling of being on top of any situation, and of sitting on top of the world. And that's the feeling of being fully alive.

14

Changing into a Winning Personality—and Leading a Fulfilling Sex Life

Since Harold has been on the Diet for Life, his personality has undergone a wonderful change.

He had always been a brilliant, charming, and witty man, but he had been shy, self-effacing, and so willing to sympathize with the other guy's viewpoint that he seldom came away with the rewards he deserved. He never lost, but he never really won. Now he goes after what he wants, knows his own worth, stands up for his rights, and wins.

He always got along with people, but he never really liked them, and preferred a good book to a good conversation. Now he finds all kinds of people interesting, goes to parties, has learned the value of the interplay of emotions and thoughts between human beings, and he treasures it.

He was a man who loved deeply and showed it, but he found it difficult to accept love. This was frustrating to those who loved him, and a source of discontent to Harold, for he wanted as much love as he could get. Now his defenses against accepting love are gone. He loves being loved, and he's loved more for it.

A free-lance writer's life is not easy. You stand alone. There's no union backing you, no corporate structure behind you, no government support. You have to fight your own battles. Harold often told me that each day was like going into an arena against a pack of hungry lions. He had his periods of anxiety, tension, depression, and of outright fear of failure and rejection. They're self-defeating emotions; they wound, cripple, and strangle the impulses of creativity and joy.

Now he has secure feelings about himself, built on a conviction of his own self-worth. He no longer sees life as an arena, but as an incomparably beautiful magic city in which each day he makes exciting discoveries about the people and the things in it, and his relationship to them. He's at the peak of his creativity—one reviewer called his last book "terrific . . . superb"—and he takes great joy in his work and in his life. When recently a radio interviewer asked him his definition of success, he replied, "Getting the most mileage out of every day." He does.

He has recovered all the rights to which a human adult is entitled: the right to feel important; to feel relaxed; to be assertive and productive; to share his life in loving intimacy with another—and, above all, the right to live his life to the fullest.

Did sound nutrition, our Diet for Life, help bring about these phenomenal changes? There's no way we can be sure, but we think so. Religions have always related the right kind of food with spiritual well-being. Myths and rituals, tracing back to the dawn of mankind, have invested certain foods with mystical properties which endowed the eater with courage, insight, virtue, sexual drive and potency, physical prowess, health, fertilty, wisdom, and even holiness. Priests and shamans may have been the pre-scientific nutritionists; and what they discovered through a primal closeness to nature, scientists may be rediscovering in their hyper-technological clinics and laboratories.

Scientific findings so far in the field of psychological nutrition are not voluminous. But there is a general recognition that the well-nourished person is better able not just to cope, but to deal well with day-by-day stresses, and to operate on a more acute emotional and intellectual level of awareness. When that happens it is not unlikely that a decided positive personality change could occur. *Man ist was er ess.* Man is what he eats.

Yet the mutations of the human psyche, for good or for evil, are far too complex to be explained solely by the food we eat or fail to eat. But food could be a factor. And the supposition is strengthened when we consider the role vitamins play in our emotional health.

Vitamins Can Improve Your Personality

It has been established that many autistic and hyperkinetic children, schizophrenics, and manic depressives have been restored to normality through nutritional therapy based essentially on the use of massive (mega) doses of vitamins B_3, C, and E. B_3 in quantities from 3,000 to 15,000 milligrams a day (the R.D.A. is 20) has been known to bring about remission of psychotic symptoms. (The mental disturbances of victims of pellagra, a vitamin-B_3-deficiency disease, parallels those of a significant number of psychotics.)

But vitamins are not magic pills. They're effective in the treatment of mental disorders only when accompanied by sound nutritional practices. Potential emotional irritants like caffeine, and food additives, colorings, and preservatives are banned from the diet. Sugar is eliminated, and a prudent balance is struck between complex carbohydrates, fats, and proteins to hinder involuntary emotional flare-ups. These dietary restrictions are bedrock elements of the Diet for Life.

Few of us, though, suffer from chronic mental disorders (and for those who do, competent medical care is mandatory). What afflicts all of us at some time to some extent are emotional states which degrade our personality, and deprive us of the inborn right to be the person we should be. Hopefully, vitamins, as part of a healthful nutritional program, like the Diet for Life, could help correct these negative emotional states and lead to a fully realized you.

In the following list, check off the negative emotional states that seem to be holding you back from self-realization (they're arranged alphabetically), and think of the joyous new you you could be without them.

VITAMINS THAT MAY HELP COUNTER
YOUR NEGATIVE EMOTIONAL STATES

Your Negative Emotional States	*Counter Vitamins*
☐ Anxiety	B_2, B_6
☐ Apathy	B_1
☐ Depression	B_1; pantothenic acid; E
☐ Dullness	B_{12}; inositol
☐ Hyperactivity	B_1; B_3
☐ Irritability	B_1; B_3
☐ Lack of appetite	C; B_3; pantothenic acid
☐ Lack of morale	B_1
☐ Lack of sales resistance (and resistance to any kind of persuasion)	B_1
☐ Lack of sense of humor	B_3
☐ Lassitude	C; B_1; B_3
☐ Malaise (feeling generally unhappy and rundown)	C
☐ Moodiness (exaggerated fluctuations in mood)	B_2; B_{12}
☐ Negative-ism ("I can't do it")	B_3
☐ Nervousness	B_1
☐ Psychosomatic aches and pains	folic acid
☐ Psychosomatic fatigue	B_1; B_2; B_6; E
☐ Psychosomatic headaches	B_3

☐ Restlessness	C
☐ Stress	B-complex vitamins; C; E
☐ Tension	B_1
☐ Uncertainty of memory	B_1, B_2; B_3; B_{12}
☐ Weepiness	C

Some Minerals Can Help Maintain Mental Health

The biochemistry of the emotions is in its infancy. Scientists have only a raw pioneering knowledge of the roles minerals play in mental health. But they have discovered that deficiencies of some minerals can induce sub-clinical mental disturbances, as shown in the following list (the minerals are arranged alphabetically):

MINERALS AND EMOTIONAL STATES

Insufficient quantities of these minerals . . .	. . . induce these emotional states
Calcium	Insomnia; nervousness; depression; irritability
Cobalt	Temper tantrums
Iodine	Sexual apathy; lassitude
Iron	Depression; emotional exhaustion; sexual apathy
Magnesium	Confusion; depression
Manganese	Sexual apathy
Phosphorus	Dullness; sexual apathy
Potassium	Emotional fatigue; depression; tension; nervousness
Silicones	Insomnia
Sodium	Emotional fatigue; depression; lassitude
Zinc	Loss of interest in learning; sexual apathy; lassitude

R.D.A.'s of the minerals listed eliminate deficiency-induced emotional states and help maintain mental health. Any sound diet, like the Diet for Life, will supply R.D.A.'s for minerals. *Caution:* Do not exceed R.D.A.'s. Excess minerals can be toxic (page 263).

When healthful foods, and the minerals they contain, are combined with your D.D.A.'s for vitamins, you could be slamming the lid on a Pandora's box of dietary-induced emotional disturbances. Free of those disturbances, you'll feel more vigorous, younger, more creative. And when you feel that way, it's time for sex.

Sex Goes On 24 Hours a Day

After his heart attack, Harold asked his cardiologist, "What about sex?"

The doctor answered, "It would be safer not to indulge."

It was chilling advice to both of us. We regarded our lovemaking, which went on for more than an hour each time, as play raised to a fine art. It was the time when the world as work and effort and striving stopped, and in some carefree outer space of the spirit we were alone in an adult playground which we created, moment by moment, from the stuff of our fantasies. Now we were afraid even to touch each other.

It was a bitter deprivation. Ours had been no ordinary love affair. It began when Harold was the editor-in-chief of a small publishing company, and I was his assistant. When I came to my desk one morning, there was a rose on it—and after that it was roses, and wine, and poetry, and stars in our eyes, and songs in our hearts, and walking on air; it was touches and glances and murmurs and kisses and the 1,001 Arabian nights of wonders we created for each other out of the commonplaces of each day. It was the second time around for each of us, and we had never even dreamed before that such love could exist. It was so beautiful. And the act of sex was its confirmation, its assertion, its culmination. And now it was replaced by fear.

But something else happened to our sex life that was even worse.

Sex is not just going to bed together.

Sex is listening to each other, touching, holding hands, smiling at each other. Sex is sharing time, ideas, pleasures, sorrows, daily chores, meals. Sex is sharing a bathroom. Sex is facing mutual problems together. Sex is facing individual problems together. Sex is facing the world together.

Sex is being honest, and loyal, and supportive. Sex is helping each other. Sex is not holding grudges. Sex is humming in the shower, washing each other's backs. Sex is touching knees in the movies. Sex is kisses. Sex is embraces. Sex is respect for each other.

Sex is sometimes saying yes when you want to say no. Sex is cuddling together at night like two pieces of a jigsaw puzzle. Sex is shopping together. Sex is thoughtfulness. Sex is the feeling of belonging but not being owned. Sex is making each other feel special.

Sex is something that goes on 24 hours a day. But on the drugs prescribed for him by his cardiologist, Harold became somebody else, and there was no sex for us *any* minute of the day. Our love affair had been the peak experience of our lives, and now it was replaced by a barren distance between us.

Then a glorious thing happened. When the Diet for Life began to work, and when he threw away the last of his drugs, he became himself again. Sex once more became part of our lives 24 hours a

day. That first time we had sex again after two dismal years, we
clung to each other, deeply desiring it would never end, and it
seemed as if it wouldn't, until suddenly, in a burst of splendor, it was
over, and we were laughing and crying at the same time, and we
knew from now on everything was going to be all right.

On the Diet for Life, Harold wanted me more than ever before—
and to have a man feel that way is one of the most wonderful experiences in a woman's life. My desire for him mounted too. And why
not? He was attractively slimmer, brimming with health and vitality,
looked 10 years younger, and behaved 30 years younger. All his
characteristics which had attracted me to him in the first place—his
charm, his brilliance, his understanding of a woman's emotional
needs, his flair for telling me how much he loved me with every
muscle of his body, his insight, were now sharpened, heightened.
Our sex appeal for each other had always been 10; now it was 10
with a long string of zeros following it.

We wondered just what in the Diet for Life had raised our lives to
this level of joy. We researched the subject, and here's what we
discovered.

The Secret of Sexual Power. . .

. . . Provided there are no physical impairments or psychological
hangups, is simple: good nutrition. The right amount of the right
foods, supplemented with the amounts of vitamins that are right for
you, manufactures hormones in sufficient quantities to strengthen
your manhood or your womanhood. Good nutrition gives you the
energy to perform often, and for long periods. It makes you look
younger, more desirable. I think—and there is some evidence to
prove it—that it causes the body to send out chemical messengers,
pheromones, the perfumes of love, that attract us to each other.
Most important, it makes us want sex—*really* want it; and when a
healthy human being really wants something, it's natural to go after
it. What man or woman doesn't love to be pursued? That's nature's
most potent aphrodisiac.

Are There Aphrodisiacs?

Love potions have been part of sexual lore from time imme-
morial. But examine them in the light of what we know now about
food, and the magic ingredient in all of them turns out to be: good
nutrition. Astonishingly, there hasn't been a love potion from an-
cient times to the present that doesn't contain one or more of the
following ingredients: garlic, shallots, onions, leeks, parsley, fish,
lean meat, poultry, fresh vegetables, mushrooms, and honey. If we

are to believe sexual lore, then most Diet-for-Life meals are love potions. And, indeed, they are, because healthful food is a tonic to both the mind and body, and the sexual urge derives from both.

But two ingredients of the Diet for Life, lecithin and vitamin E, have gained a reputation as specific aphrodisiacs. Let's see if the reputation is justified.

Is Lecithin for Lovers?

With his morning vitamin cocktail, and with his after-lunch and after-dinner vitamins, Harold takes a total of 2,400 grains of soy lecithin.

He added it to his diet for a trio of reasons. It's supposed to act much like a soap, emulsify fats, and wash them out of the arteries. It's said to assist in the production of H.D.L.'s which dispose of excess arterial cholesterol. And it's known to contain substantial quantities of choline, which is essential to fat metabolism, and of inositol, which is claimed to reduce blood-cholesterol deposits.

He didn't add it to his diet because he thought it was a sexual stimulant. Yet one widely read nutritionist thinks it is, in the sense that it's a rejuvenant, a substance that turns back the aging clock. If this claim has any validity at all, it's probably based on the following explanation.

Lecithin is present in every cell of the body, with the highest concentrations in the organs most essential to life—heart, liver, kidneys, muscle, nerves, and brain (less water, 30% of the brain is composed of lecithin). A lecithin deficiency could diminish physical and mental well-being, as aging does, with a consequent decline in sexual drive. The restoration of lecithin levels throughout the body could create the effect of feeling younger, with a consequent boost to the libido. Only in this roundabout way can lecithin be for lovers.

Can Vitamin E Improve Sexual Health?

This vitamin has long been been popularly regarded as *the* sex vitamin since it is in many ways directly related to the sex function.

Deprivation of vitamin E produces sterility. Testicles of laboratory animals shrivel on vitamin E-deficient diets, and sex-hormone levels in both sexes significantly decline. (Vitamin E is essential to the manufacture of these hormones in the body.) Vitamin E can help correct irregular menstrual cycles, and help relieve the hot flushes, irritability, and headaches of menopause.

But among humans, vitamin E has no effect on frigidity (sexual apathy and failure to achieve orgasm in a female) or on impotence (lack, infrequency, or shortness of duration of an erection). Frigidity (an ugly word) is probably caused by clumsy lovers, psychological straitjackets, moral inhibitions, and personal preference (more than 50% of American women, according to a recent poll, *don't like* sex). Impotence can be caused by diabetes, vascular problems affecting the genitalia, multiple sclerosis, endocrine dysfunctions, certain prostate conditions, spinal cord injuries or diseases, and alcoholism; but more than eight times out of 10, the roots are psychological.

There is no evidence, either, that vitamin E can improve sexual performance.

But vitamin E does prevent the oxidation of fats in cells (a process much like oil going rancid), which is a principal cause of aging. And vitamin E helps get more oxygen to your tissues, which can make you feel as if you were going through the day with an aqualung on your back. So with aging slowed down, and oxygen power surging through your body, you're likely to feel younger and more vigorous than you felt before you began to take vitamin E. And youth and vigor usually spell "sex." Only in this indirect way can vitamin E be regarded as improving your sexual health.

What About Wine and Sex?

In vino veritas—"under the influence of wine, the truth comes out." If you truly desire sex, wine helps.

Wine is an option on the Diet for Life because it's a delight to the palate, a nonpareil promoter of social conviviality and a sense of physical well-being, a healthful food with possible antibiotic qualities, an antagonist of heart attack (alcohol may take part in the production of H.D.L.'s), and a passport from the dining room to the bedroom.

It's not the alcohol by itself that increases sexual desire (vodka, which is pure alcohol and water, has a deadening effect on the sexual impulse), but the interplay of alcohol with certain chemicals, synergens, in the brew. Some wines contain these synergens in the right sex-stimulating proportions; some don't. In our experience, the wines that don't, include all whites, except Champagne, and all sweet wines. The wines that do—and these are the ones that grace our dinner table most often—are dry reds, the drier the better.

Just how much wine to drink to heighten sexual desire and performance must be determined by trial and error. Too little wine—and nothing happens. Too much wine—and nothing happens (desire is aroused, but bed is for sleeping only). We never drink more than a glass of wine each *with food*. That's important because the food slows down the ingestion of the alcohol *cum* synergens; and the slower they feed into the bloodstream, the greater the sexual stimulus. Never gulp wine. Sip for sex.

Wine presents no conflict between sex and slimness. Alcohol contributes about 7 calories a gram, as compared to 9 for fat; but don't let that frighten you. The amount of alcohol in wine is small (ordinarily 10% to 12% by volume); and eight ounces of wine contribute only 168 calories. Besides, when wine leads to prolonged sex, you can use up those calories as fast as if you were jogging. You'll also be happy to know that there's no biochemical pathway by which alcohol can be converted into fat. (How about beer guzzlers, with their big bellies? They *eat* too much, and they eat too much *salted* food.)

Wine has this additional attraction: you linger over it. The dinner meal, the second most intimate act of our day, lasts longer. Wine prolongs the pleasure of two kindred spirits blending into one. And that's the perfect prelude to healthful sex.

A vôtre santé!

Dining for Love

You can't get sexy over oatmeal; but you can over foods that turn you on. There are so many haute cuisine dishes in the Diet for Life which call to our minds Strauss waltzes, and candlelight, and gleaming silver, and two hearts beating in three-quarter time.

At our dinner table, I enhance the basic romantic appeal of my dishes with flowers, and beautiful tableware and napery. The food is presented in artistically colorful patterns. There are soft lights; and sentimental music, played just above the level of audibility, touches us softly. The ambiance of eating is just as much a part of the joy of the Diet for Life as the food itself.

Then as we eat and sip our wine, a magic curtain descends over the business of the day. Now there is nothing in the world except the two of us. This is the time to talk about ourselves, who we are, who we're trying to be. Our conversation is a gentle excursion into each other's dreams and aspirations. We understand each other, accept each other, help each other, draw closer.

We listen to each other with open hearts. And with each heartbeat we assure each other in myriad subtle ways that no one else is more important in the whole wide world. We feed on each other's warmth. We touch. We kiss. We are two people who love each other, and who are very much in love.

Sex is built on love. Our dinner is a love feast. When dinner is over and we desire each other, we don't have sex—we make love.

The Diet for Life was created out of love. The Diet for Life creates love.

Manhattan
Summer, 1980

Sources of Some Favored Ingredients

Low-Sodium Baking Powder, manufactured by Chicago Dietetic Supply, Inc.; LaGrange, Ill. 60525

Date Powder, manufactured by Sunshine Valley Foods; Canoga Park, Calif. 91304

Smoked Yeast, manufactured by Sovex, Inc.; Collegedale, Tenn. 37315

Wheat or Rice Allgrane Wafers (unsalted), manufactured by Devonshire Melba Corporation; Carlstadt, N.J. 07072

Chicken of the Sea dietetic-pack chunk-white albacore tuna in water, no salt added, packed by Van Camp Sea Food Co.; San Diego, Calif. 92121

Fearn's non-fat dry milk, manufactured by Fearn Soya Foods; Melrose Park, Ill. 60160

Cafix (coffee substitute). U.S. Importers: Richter Brothers, Inc.; Carlstadt, N.J. 07072

Carob, manufactured by El Molino Mills, Inc.; P. O. Box 2250, City of Industry, Calif. 91746

Norwegian Dietetic Brisling Sardines, no salt or oil added, packed by Season Products Corp. A/S, Stavanger, Norway. Distributed by Season Products Corp.; Irvington, N.J. 07111

Matzo-Thins, no salt, sugar, shortening, spices, or artificial sweeteners added, manufactured by Manischewitz Company; P. O. Box 484A, Jersey City, N.J. 07303

Spice Islands Chili Con Carne Seasoning, manufactured by Specialty Brands, Inc.; San Francisco, Calif. 94133.

Grated Sap Sago Cheese, imported by Emmental Cheese Corp.; 175 Clearbrook Road, Elmsford, N.Y. 10523

Recipe Index

Subject Index